Think Outside The Medicine Cabinet

A Comprehensive Workbook on
Integrating Medical and Behavioral Health Strategies
to Manage Chronic Pain Effectively

Glenn L. Banks
Creator of SHRP

Contents

Acknowledgements

"I am grateful to my Heavenly Father and His Son Jesus Christ for the precious gift of life and the opportunities to grow in knowledge and serve others.

My heart is full of love and gratitude toward my wife, Stacey, and our precious children - Laina, Alexis, Haley, and Shawn. I cannot thank you enough for supporting me through challenges and triumphs in my work as a helping professional. I have striven to be the best husband and father I could be. Your presence has brought joy, comfort, and entertainment to my life.

I want to thank my mother who has been a saving grace in this life. She has always seen in me what I could not see. She has been there to encourage me when I felt lonely. She sacrificed for me when I needed it.

To all my mentors and fellow professionals who have influenced and supported me throughout my professional journey, particularly Delbert Billman, Reed Robinson, Robert Wilson, Juliette Beeman, Suzanne Northey, Jason Frizzell, Barbara Dal Monte, and Adam Lundberg, I am grateful for your guidance and encouragement.

Finally, I extend my sincere gratitude to all those who have experienced the struggles of living with chronic pain. It has been an honor to learn from your courage and resilience, and I am grateful for the privilege of accompanying you on this journey."

Glenn Banks

"Pain is not in your head, and the solution is not in your body."

-Dr. Howard Schubiner, MD. Physician, researcher, and author specializing in the treatment of chronic pain.

Introduction

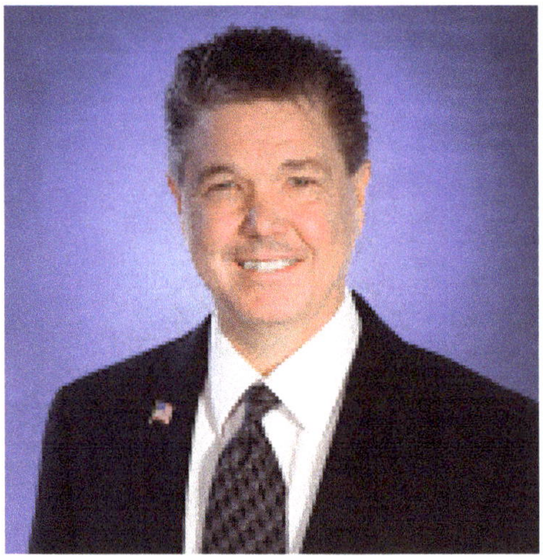

"Throughout my career, I've assisted individuals from diverse backgrounds by providing counseling services to families, couples, and individuals. I've worked as a mobile crisis team member, prison and jail psychology associate therapist, clinical care planner for Seriously Mentally Ill (SMI) clinics, and an SMI evaluator.

However, my experience at a chronic pain clinic made me realize that despite my knowledge of the brain's role in regulating thoughts, emotions, and behaviors, I lacked the expertise to fully support my patients. Witnessing their distress and despair propelled me to deepen my understanding of the brain and its functions. I thought, "There has to be answers out there!"

Three significant revelations inspired me to write this book. Firstly, I became a Certified Trauma Professional to serve the 20% of patients with chronic pain who exhibit trauma symptoms. During my certification, I learned that the brain's primary function is to keep us safe, leading me to change my approach to chronic pain counseling and focus on promoting safety in all aspects of my patient's lives.

My second revelation occurred during a discussion with a family member who is a pain doctor. He introduced me to the "Wind-up Effect" or Central Sensitization. This effect stabilizes chronic pain signals, even when patients comply with treatment plans. The brain does this to protect us and give us a sense of safety.

Finally, by implementing the Bio-Psycho-Social-Spiritual Pain (BPSS-P) approach in counseling sessions with patients suffering from chronic pain, I realized that meeting their fundamental human needs, such as the need for spirituality, belonging, variety, importance, and basic needs, effectively mitigates the "wind-up effect" in the brain. This results in much less chronic pain signaling and provides relief of symptoms while promoting safety.

These revelations, with my past experiences in the helping professions, energized me to develop the Strategic Harm Reduction Plan (SHRP). Since its implementation, I've seen remarkable progress in patients who have dedicated their time and effort to following the plan and significantly reduced their chronic pain.

My primary mission is to support individuals with chronic pain and other conditions, helping them feel safe in all areas of their lives. If you or someone you know is struggling with chronic pain, I highly encourage you to explore the benefits of the SHRP. By following the plan, you can witness remarkable strides in managing chronic pain more effectively and taking control of your life."

Don't hesitate - what do you or anyone have to lose? Pain?!

Glenn L. Banks

“

All people occasionally stumble across the truth, but most pick themselves up and continue as if nothing had happened.”

-Winston Churchill

AN OLD SIOUX LEGEND...

In ancient times, the Creator wanted to hide something from the humans until they were ready to see it. He gathered all the other creatures of creation to ask their advice.

The eagle said, "Give it to me and I will take it to the highest mountain in all the land," but the Creator said,
"No, one day they will conquer the mountain and find it."

The salmon said, "Leave it with me and I will hide it at the very bottom of the ocean," but the Creator said,
"No, for humans are explorers at heart, and one day they will go there too."

The buffalo said, "I will take it and bury it in the very heart of the great plains." But the Creator said, "No, for one day even the skin of the Earth will be ripped open, and they will find it there."

The creatures of creation were stumped, but an old blind mole spoke up. "Why don't you put it inside them — that's the very last place they'll look."

The Creator said, "It is done."

"Chronic pain is not a choice. It's not a weakness. It's a condition that deserves to be taken seriously."

-Cindy Steinberg, National Director of Policy and Advocacy

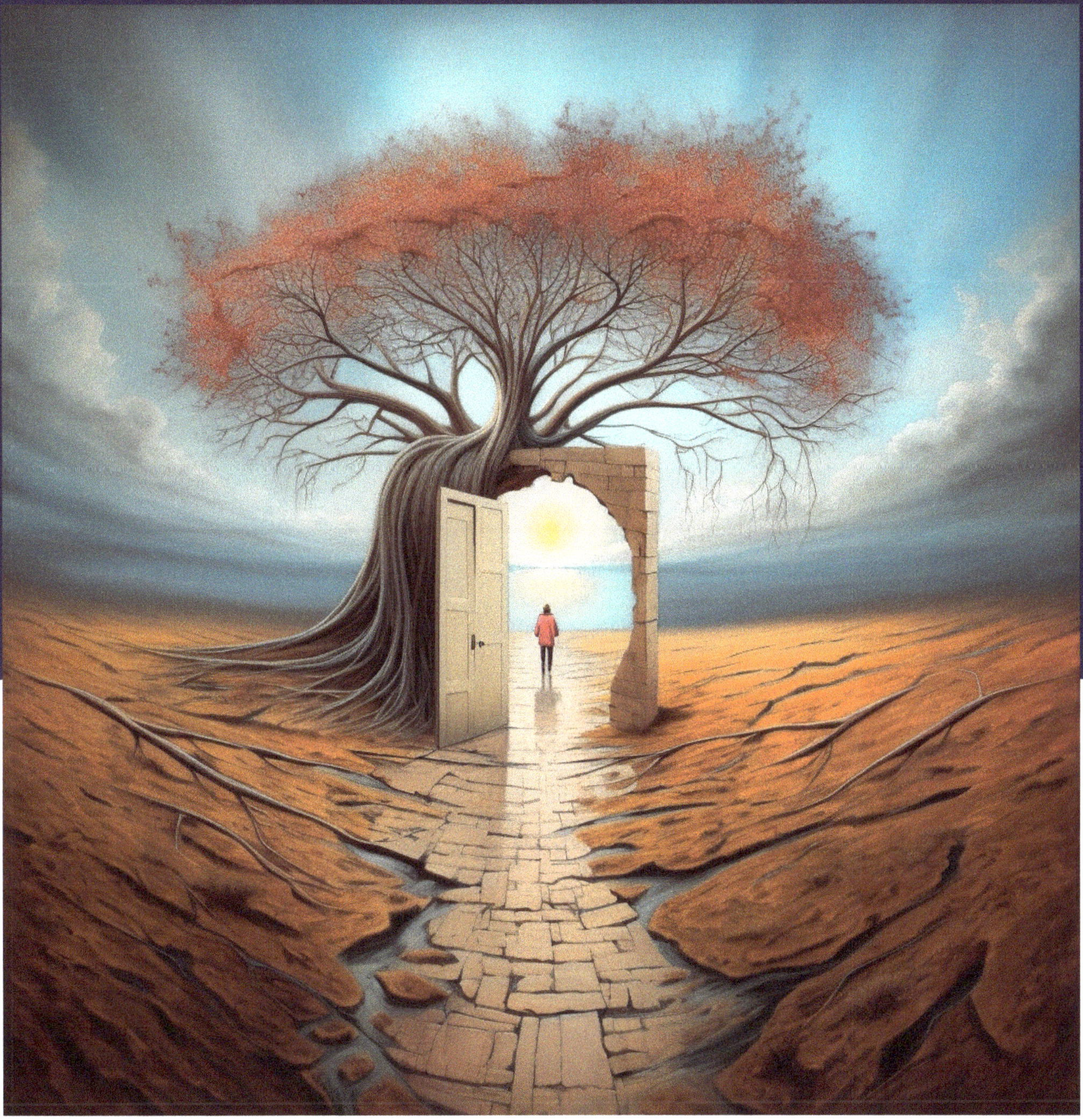

Chapter One

Breaking The Stigma

The old Sioux legend above refers to the belief that the Creator, or Great Spirit, had hidden a sacred stone with extraordinary powers somewhere on Earth. The Creator believed humans were not ready to possess this power and kept it hidden until the right time. Eventually, the Creator decided to put this power inside humans so that they could access it and use it for good.

This legend is often interpreted as a metaphor for the idea that humans have the potential for greatness and possess the power to achieve extraordinary things but don't know where to find it.

The power to change one's situation and improve a person's quality of life is within everyone. By embracing alternative therapies, such as physical therapy, acupuncture, mindfulness meditation, art therapy, and so much more, a person can regain control over chronic pain and reduce their reliance on prescription drugs.

These proven alternative modalities provide individuals with the tools to tap into their inner strength and facilitate their healing journey. The power to transform one's life is not external but rather lies within every human being.

With a comprehensive approach, you can explore inventive solutions that cater to your unique needs, eventually attaining relief from chronic pain. Instead of settling for unwanted side effects and the possibility of dependence or addiction, you can embrace evidence-based treatments that have been verified to decrease chronic pain and enhance overall well-being.

Your skepticism is understood. You might have heard recommendations such as "just breathe better" or "take a warm bath" and pondered if there's more to it. The truth is, there is much more. This book will steer you through evidence-based treatments, providing you with a better comprehension of your chronic pain and the myriad solutions at your disposal.

Discovering the perfect blend of therapies may demand some time and effort, but the prospective benefits are life-altering. Refuse to permit chronic pain to govern your life any longer. Say farewell to skepticism and welcome to some relief. What do you stand to lose? Pain. Here is a typical patient with a chronic pain experience:

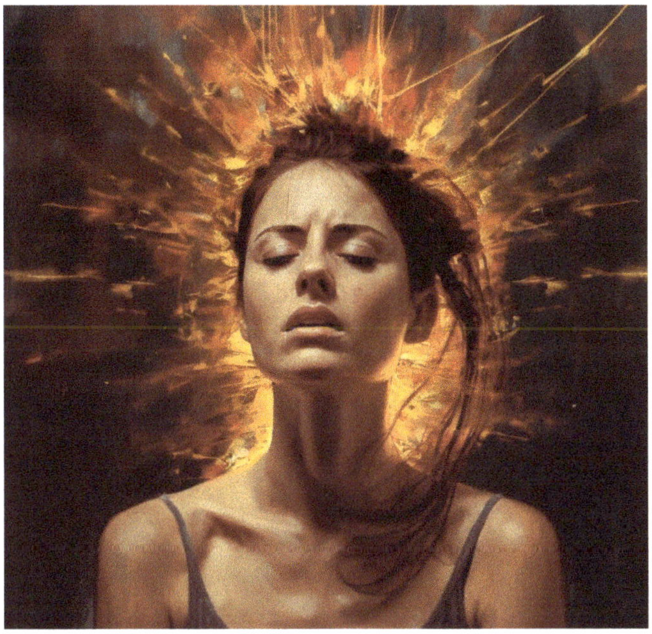

"Sarah had been struggling with chronic back pain for what felt like an eternity. She had seen more doctors than she could count, each promising a solution, but offering nothing more than pain medication or injections that did little to alleviate her constant discomfort.

Despite her many visits, she couldn't help but feel like she was just another case, shuffled through the medical system without a second thought. What was worse, she had grown used to the incredulous looks and skeptical questions from her doctors, pharmacists, counselors, and even her family members and friends, who all wondered if she was exaggerating her symptoms, or worse, seeking out opioids for recreational use.

The irony was not lost on Sarah. She had always been taught to trust doctors and that they knew what was best for her, but here she was, treated with suspicion and doubt. As the years passed, Sarah's frustration with the medical system grew. She felt like she was constantly having to defend herself and her pain, instead of being offered the help she desperately needed."

Chronic pain is more than just a physical sensation; it is a complex and multifaceted experience that involves physical, emotional, and psychological factors."

-Beth Darnall

The quote by Beth Darnall, a pain psychologist, and researcher at Stanford University, emphasizes the extensive nature of chronic pain and highlights the importance of addressing not only the physical symptoms but also the emotional and psychological aspects of pain management.

Research has demonstrated that chronic pain frequently has a substantial impact on an individual's day-to-day activities, interpersonal connections, and overall well-being.

Achieving successful treatment outcomes requires a holistic approach that considers all facets of an individual's chronic pain experience, which is essential.

Understanding the experiences of patients with chronic pain when interacting with medical professionals is necessary for several reasons.

- Firstly, it sheds light on the numerous challenges and obstacles that many individuals with chronic pain encounter when seeking medical treatment. The stigma and skepticism that surrounds chronic pain is real and can make it challenging for people to receive appropriate care and support, which can lead to feelings of frustration, and hopelessness, and can even worsen their pain.[1]
- Secondly, having a better understanding of the experiences of patients with chronic pain can help healthcare providers to develop more comprehensive and compassionate approaches to treating chronic pain. For instance, doctors can work to avoid stigmatizing patients with chronic pain and develop treatment plans that consider the physical, emotional, and psychological aspects of pain management.[2]
- Finally, raising awareness about the difficulties faced by people with chronic pain can help to minimize the social isolation and misunderstanding that they experience. This can lead to increased public support for initiatives in advancing research into more effective treatments for chronic pain and improving pain management overall.[3]

This book aims to raise awareness and promote a deeper understanding of chronic pain and emphasizes the significance of this understanding for healthcare providers, patients, and society. In addition to increasing awareness, this book offers practical advice, and a guide for patients with chronic pain to navigate the complex and personal world of chronic pain and become effective advocates for their needs.

This book seeks to engage readers by offering valuable insights and perspectives that can help healthcare providers better understand the needs of patients with chronic pain and develop more extensive and compassionate approaches to pain management.

It also seeks to guide healthcare providers on how to avoid stigmatizing patients with chronic pain and develop treatment plans that address the physical, emotional, and psychological aspects of chronic pain.

By offering these tools, this book can empower patients and healthcare providers to work together towards improving pain management and advancing research into effective treatments. In essence, this book is an ongoing project, that will never truly be finished due to the dynamic nature of chronic pain.

As the field evolves, this book aims to catalyze meaningful dialogue and effectual transformation of the care and support of individuals experiencing chronic pain within the healthcare system and society.

Quotes To Spark
Thought And Discussion

"Chronic pain is a thief, stealing time, relationships, and joy."

-Anonymous

"The reality of chronic pain is that it affects every aspect of your life. It's not just a physical sensation, it's an emotional and psychological one as well."

-Nicole Hemmenway, chronic pain advocate and author

"Chronic pain is like a guest who never leaves. It's always there, lurking in the background, waiting for an opportunity to take over."

-Glenn Banks

"Chronic pain can deprive individuals of their time, robbing them of precious moments that ought to be savored and enjoyed."

-John Durbin, Chronic Pain Advocate

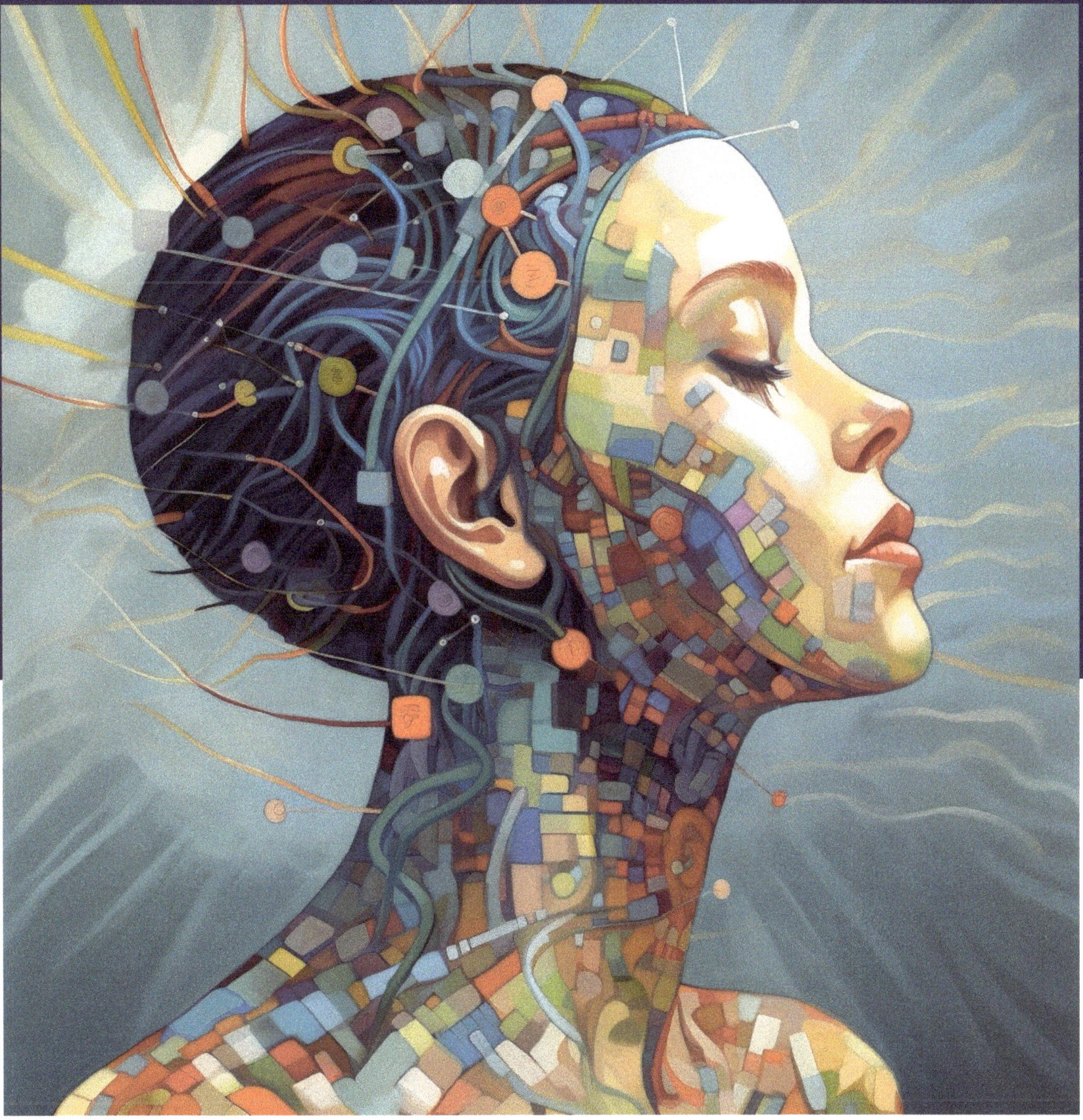

Chapter Two

Decoding Pain

Pain is not solely a physical sensation but also an emotional experience that significantly impacts a person's quality of life. Coping with pain can be challenging, but it's meaningful to recognize that it's not an enemy to be vanquished or a punishment to be endured.

> ***Chronic pain is not an enemy or punishment...it is only a signal!***

Pain is a signal from the body that demands attention. Although it can be highly unpleasant, pain serves a vital purpose, and it should not be considered a sign of weakness to seek relief from it. A curious and open approach toward pain can facilitate the discovery of various treatment options and strategies, resulting in more successful personal pain management. We will delve into two types of pain: acute and chronic pain.

Acute pain is typically short-lived, caused by tissue damage or injury, and serves as a warning signal to protect the body. It's characterized by a sharp or intense sensation localized to a specific area. It usually resolves within a few weeks or months with medication, physical therapy, or other interventions targeting the underlying cause. It's essential to comprehend that the brain's natural protective process continues even in chronic pain that may persist for years.

Chronic pain is a multifaceted medical and psychological condition that is caused by structural changes in the nervous system, specifically called, "Central Sensitization" or "Wind-up Effect" of pain signals. This can occur due to various factors, such as ongoing inflammation or nerve damage.

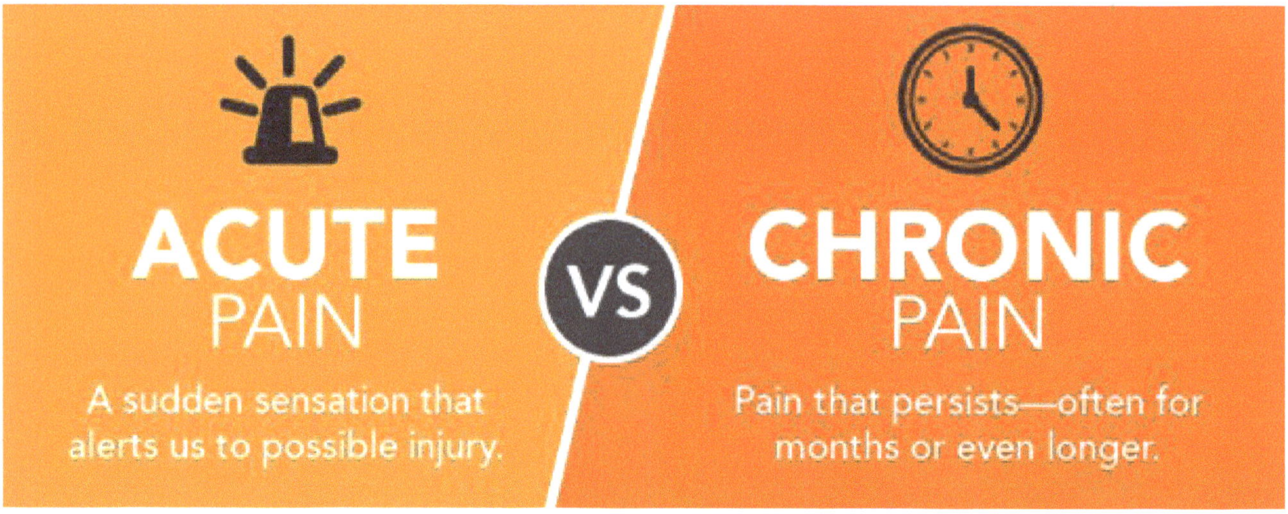

Courtesy of www.health.mil

When the brain perceives a threat, it releases stress hormones, adrenaline, and neurotransmitters like norepinephrine and dopamine. These chemicals increase alertness, attention, and focus to enable the body to react to the perceived threat, by fighting, fleeing, or freezing.

Once the perceived threat subsides, the body returns to its normal state through the "relaxation response." However, when acute pain is perceived as a constant threat, the body's "fight, flight, or freeze" response is repeatedly triggered. If not effectively managed, acute pain can then escalate, significantly impacting a person's quality of life and structurally changing the person's brain. Therefore, addressing the physical and psychological aspects of acute pain is important to help the brain feel more secure and alleviate the perceived threat, which is the number one purpose: to keep us safe.

When we say that the number one purpose of the brain is to keep us safe, we are referring to the fundamental role of the brain in ensuring our survival, well-being, and protection from harm. This perspective emphasizes the brain's evolutionary function of detecting and responding to potential environmental threats and dangers.

Safety can be defined as a state or condition in which one senses freedom from harm, danger, or risk. It encompasses physical safety, emotional well-being, and psychological security. Safety involves the absence or mitigation of threats, the presence of protective measures, and the ability to navigate the environment to minimize harm.

The brain's role in maintaining safety involves several interconnected processes, including:

- ***Perception and Sensing:*** The brain continuously processes sensory information from the environment to detect potential threats or changes that may pose risks to our safety. It processes inputs from our senses (such as sight, hearing, and touch) and interprets them to identify potential dangers or opportunities for safety.
- ***Risk Assessment and Decision-Making:*** The brain evaluates and assesses the level of risk associated with different stimuli and situations. It considers past experiences, learned associations, and the current context to make decisions that prioritize safety. This includes assessing the potential consequences of actions and making choices that minimize risks.

- ***Response and Adaptation:*** When the brain perceives a threat or danger, it initiates a series of physiological and behavioral responses to protect us. These responses can include fight-or-flight reactions, stress responses, heightened vigilance, and the activation of neural circuits associated with survival instincts. The brain also can adapt and learn from experiences to improve future responses to potential threats.
- ***Regulation of Bodily Functions:*** The brain oversees the regulation of bodily functions essential for maintaining safety and well-being. This includes maintaining homeostasis, regulating heart rate, and breathing, coordinating motor skills, and managing the release of hormones and neurotransmitters associated with stress, emotions, and risk assessment.

While the brain's primary function is to keep us safe, it also encompasses other complex cognitive processes, emotions, and functions contributing to our overall human experience. These include perception, cognition, creativity, social interactions, and more. However, the drive for safety and self-preservation remains the foundational purpose of the brain's functioning.

It's important to note that safety varies across individuals, cultures, and contexts. What constitutes safety for one person may differ from another. Additionally, the brain's pursuit of safety does not necessarily imply all risks are dangerous or we must live a completely sheltered existence. It involves balancing and managing risks, seeking opportunities, and maintaining our well-being in a dynamic and ever-changing world. In the case of chronic pain, the brain continues after six to eight months of continuous pain signaling on average to perceive a threat, even without ongoing tissue damage, injury, or a real threat. Consequently, the "fight, flight, or freeze" response may remain activated, leading to adverse physical and mental health effects over time, known again as the "Wind-up effect."

Managing chronic pain, therefore, requires a comprehensive and integrated approach that addresses both the physical and psychological aspects of the condition. Let's illustrate with an imagined story:

"As Judy peacefully strolls through the dense woods during her two-hour hike, she suddenly catches sight of a shaking bush in the distance. In a fraction of a second, her brain swiftly processes numerous bits of information, interpreting the bush's movement as a possible threat. This prompts her body's stress response system to spring into action, triggering the release of adrenaline and other stress hormones.

Judy instantaneously experiences a quickened heart rate, accelerated breathing, and tense muscles, preparing her for the instinctive response of fight, flight, or freeze.

Approaching the bush, Judy couldn't see what was causing the movement. Her brain was now in overdrive, trying to gather more information and assess the situation to determine if there was a real danger. The brain's way of sensing danger and safety is to calculate answers to important questions. Is it a bear, a squirrel, or just the wind? The lack of clarity only heightened her anxiety and physical response.

Eventually, Judy cautiously approached the bush and discovered that it was just a bird perched on a branch, causing it to shake as it took flight. With this new information, her brain signaled to her body's stress response system to stand down, and her heart rate and breathing momentarily returned to normal, along with her muscle tension."

The brain's ability to rapidly respond to potential threats, even without complete information, is remarkable and can occur numerous times daily. This illustrates how our brains trigger the stress response system, preparing our bodies for action, even when the perceived threat is insignificant.[4]

But let's review this imagined story from a different perspective:

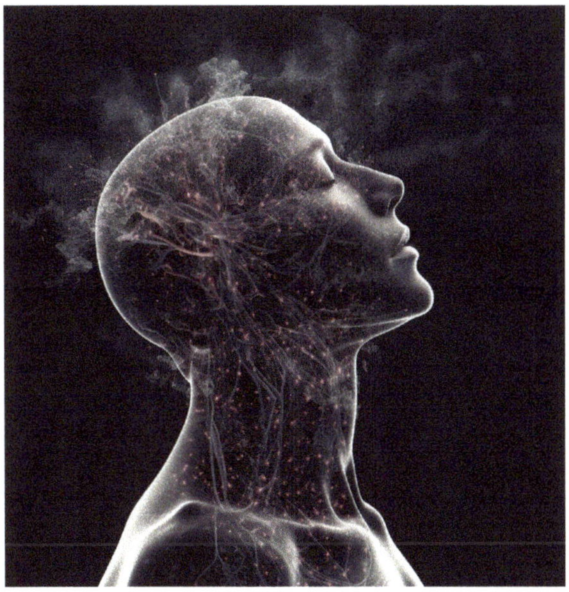

"Due to Judy's previous experience during her hike, where she witnessed a shaking bush and had concerns about a potential bear nearby (despite never encountering one), she developed a heightened sense of hyper-vigilance. This persistent state of anxiety keeps her constantly on edge, even in the absence of any immediate danger. As a result, Judy remains in a constant state of heightened alertness when she goes on any hike, or anything similar, ensuring that she is always prepared for potential threats."

Living with chronic pain can be likened to Judy's situation where the brain keeps receiving pain signals despite the absence of an immediate threat or the healing of the initial damage or injury. The continuous activation of the body's stress response system can cause several physical and psychological symptoms. Chronic pain can induce persistent stress, depression, and anxiety, which can exacerbate the body's stress response system, even if the patient is adhering to their chronic pain treatment plan.

As a result of the ongoing "Wind-up effect," individuals experiencing chronic pain may develop a range of physical symptoms, such as increased heart rate, blood pressure, respiration, muscle tension, digestive issues, and a weakened immune system. [5]

These symptoms can have a significant impact on their quality of life, making it crucial to address chronic pain as early as possible. By implementing an effective treatment and management plan, such as the Strategic Harm Reduction Plan (SHRP) outlined in this book, individuals with chronic pain can improve their daily functioning and reduce the negative impact of chronic pain on their body and mind.

Let's summarize and offer a perspective that clarifies the information provided.

The experience of pain is a natural response of the brain to injury or damage, serving as a protective mechanism for the body. However, chronic pain that extends beyond the anticipated healing period can have a significant impact on an individual's daily life and requires medical and behavioral health interventions, irrespective of their treatment adherence.

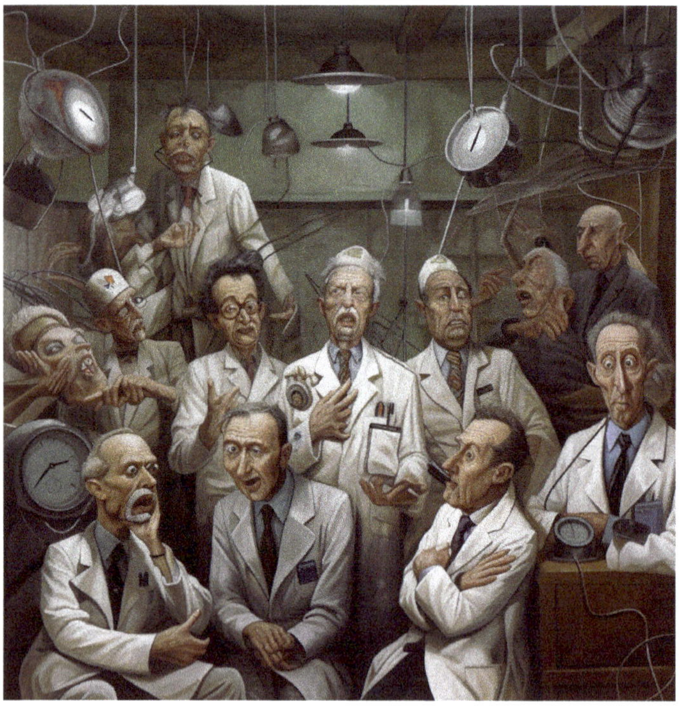

While innovative medical treatments are available, the conventional medical model usually cannot adequately address the complex mental health needs of those with chronic pain. It is essential to recognize that chronic pain involves physical, emotional, psychological, and social factors that necessitate a comprehensive and multidisciplinary approach to treatment [6]

According to the medical model, chronic pain is a physical phenomenon that entails structural changes in the nervous system and altered neurophysiological processes. However, this model also acknowledges that psychological and social factors can impact chronic pain. Therefore, even the medical community advocates for a multi-disciplinary approach to pain management that encompasses pharmacological and non-pharmacological interventions.[7]

The phrase "medical community advocates" suggests that the medical community endorses and promotes a comprehensive approach to pain management. It considers the physical, psychological, and social aspects of chronic pain. This approach involves a range of interventions, including pharmacological treatments, physical therapy, and psychological therapies, such as behavioral health interventions.

Advocating in the context of healthcare means, "To actively promote and support a specific approach or treatment as the most effective or appropriate way to address a particular condition or problem".

However, a study published in the Journal of General Internal Medicine in 2018 found that ***only 8%*** of patients with chronic pain received treatment that adhered to the bio-psycho-social model. This indicates a significant discrepancy between the endorsement of the model and its practical implementation[8]

Another study published in the Journal of Pain Research revealed that most medical providers lack education and training in non-pharmacological pain management methods, leading to a greater reliance on pharmacological therapies, which may not align with the comprehensive approach advocated by the medical model.[9] There are several potential explanations as to why physicians utilizing the medical model for chronic pain may not advocate for a multidimensional approach to pain management.

One possible factor is a lack of training or resources in non-pharmacological pain management interventions. Research published in the Journal of Pain Research indicates that numerous medical providers lack sufficient education and training in non-pharmacological pain management methods, resulting in a greater reliance on pharmacological therapies.[10]

Another potential barrier to advocating for a multidisciplinary approach to pain management is a lack of insurance coverage for non-pharmacological interventions. In a survey of primary care physicians, nearly 80% reported that insurance coverage for non-pharmacological pain management approaches was a significant barrier to their use[11]

Cultural bias towards the medical model in healthcare may also contribute to a reluctance to advocate for non-pharmacological interventions. A study published in the Journal of General Internal Medicine found that physicians may be more likely to prescribe opioids for pain management when they perceive their patients as having lower levels of social support or when they feel uncomfortable discussing non-pharmacological interventions.[12]

Finally, individual physician beliefs and practices may also play a role. In a survey of pain management physicians, attitudes towards non-pharmacological interventions varied widely, with some physicians expressing skepticism about the effectiveness of these approaches.[13]

Frankly, some physicians' skepticism regarding patients' compliance with non-pharmacological pain management interventions is based on genuine reasons and comprehensible.

To illustrate...

Imagine a health-conscious individual visiting their doctor for a routine check-up. During the consultation, the doctor asks about the patient's exercise habits, and the person confidently replies that they exercise at least five times a week.

The doctor then asks about their diet, specifically if they consume enough fruits and vegetables, and the person responds positively.

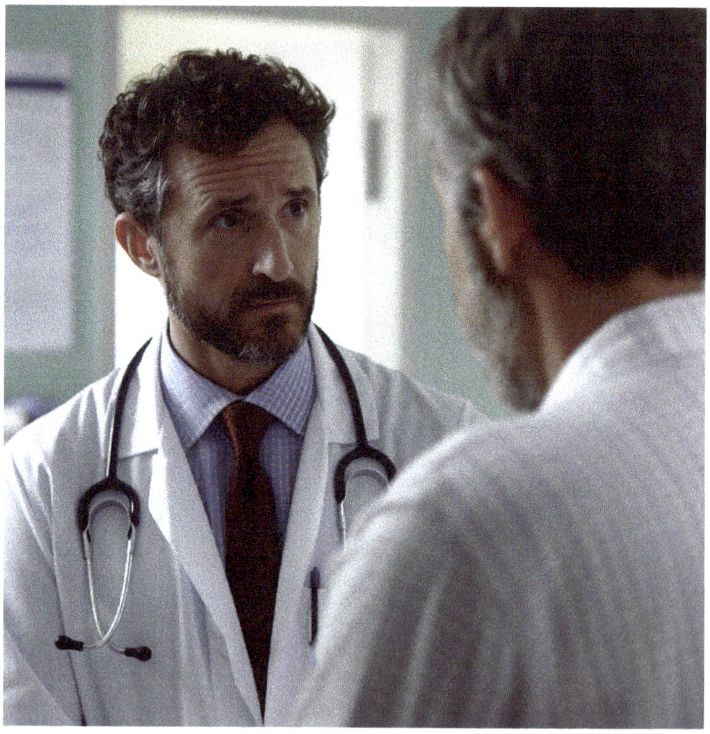

However, as the doctor examines the patient's chest, he notices a pack of cigarettes in the patient's shirt pocket. The doctor expresses surprise and points out the risks of smoking. The patient shrugs and defends their habit by saying, "Everyone has their vices."

This common scenario emphasizes the importance of addressing the disconnect between what a patient reports and what healthcare providers believe. It underscores the need for healthcare practitioners to possess knowledge and skills in non-pharmacological pain management techniques and embrace an interdisciplinary approach to pain management.

Encouraging and cultivating such healthcare practitioners is imperative in providing effective care for patients experiencing pain.

Quotes To Spark
Thought And Discussion

"The good physician treats the disease; the great physician treats the patient who has the disease."

-William Osler

"The best doctor in the world is the veterinarian. He can't ask his patients what is the matter-he's got to just know."

-Will Rogers

"The doctor of the future will give no medication but will interest his patients in the care of the human frame, diet and in the cause and prevention of disease."

-Thomas Edison

"The greatest mistake in the treatment of diseases is that there are physicians for the body and physicians for the soul, although the two cannot be separated."

-Plato

"Pain is not in your head, and the solution is not in your body."

-Dr. Howard Schubiner, MD. He is a physician, researcher, and author who specializes in the treatment of chronic pain.

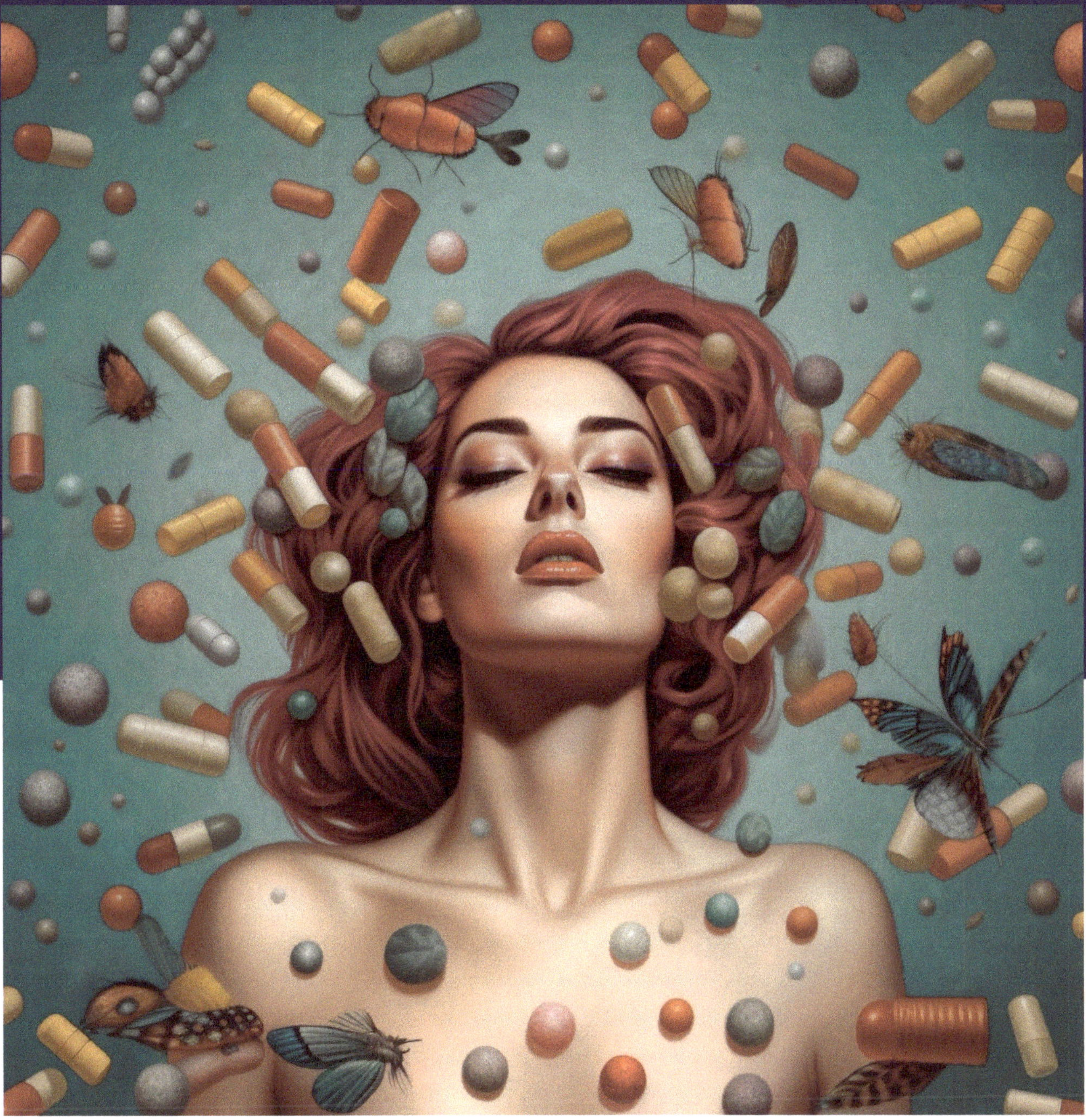

Chapter Three

Try Something Radical!

What a crazy idea! Imagine the irony. Who would have thought that chronic pain could be managed without relying so much on popping pills? But wait, it can get even crazier!?

By adopting a comprehensive, multidisciplinary approach to pain management that includes non-medical interventions, people experience better outcomes and avoid those pesky side effects. It's almost too radical to believe, right? It is time to try something radical! Maybe, let's...

"THINK OUTSIDE THE MEDICINE CABINET!"

The conventional medical model for managing chronic pain typically includes medications like non-steroidal anti-inflammatory drugs (NSAIDs), opioids, antidepressants, and anticonvulsants, as well as interventional procedures like injections and surgeries.

Nevertheless, there is a growing recognition that a one-dimensional medical approach is not sufficient to effectively address most chronic pain sufferers.

To address the multifaceted nature of chronic pain and provide more effective treatment options, it is imperative to adopt a broad-based approach that considers not only the physical symptoms but also the psychological, social, and spiritual aspects of the condition.

To achieve optimal management of chronic pain, healthcare providers and patients must prioritize the integration of three fundamental components, referred to here as the "SHRP Approach". It includes neuropsychological education, trauma-informed care, and the Biological-Psychological-Social-Spiritual Pain (BPSS-P) approach.

Integrating these components into a single comprehensive model, SHRP, not only lessens chronic pain but empowers patients to exercise control of their bodies and minds, ultimately improving their overall life experience.

This approach lessens dependence on potentially hazardous pharmacological therapies and promotes a more joyful and healthier lifestyle for individuals living with chronic pain.

Several studies suggest that a multidisciplinary approach to chronic pain management, which includes non-medical interventions, may be more effective than relying solely on medication or interventional procedures. Therefore, it is important to incorporate SHRP into the management of chronic pain to achieve the best possible outcomes.

Here are a few examples:

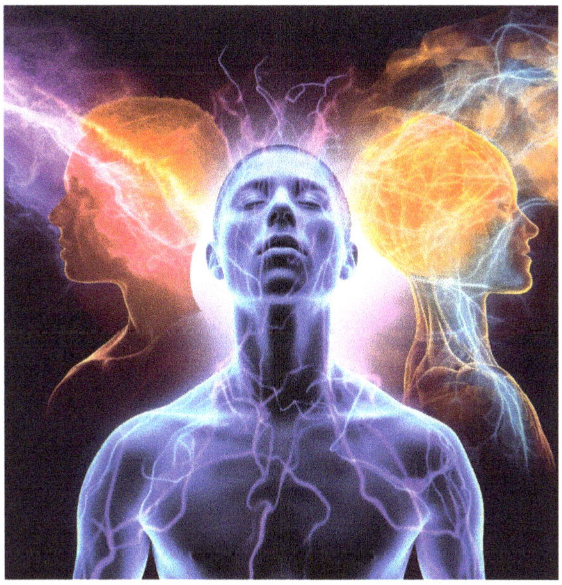

- A study published in the Journal of Pain found that patients who received multidisciplinary pain treatment, which included physical therapy, psychological interventions, and medication management, reported greater improvements in pain, physical functioning, and quality of life compared to those who received only medication management or physical therapy alone. (https://www.jpain.org/article/S1526-5900(09)00738-8/fulltext).
- A systematic review published in the Annals of Internal Medicine found that multidisciplinary pain programs that include physical therapy, psychological interventions, and other non-medical treatments are more effective than usual care in improving pain, physical function, and quality of life in patients with chronic pain. (https://www.ncbi.nlm.nih.gov/pmc/articles/PMC5548009/).
- A survey conducted by the American Chronic Pain Association found that patients who participated in multidisciplinary pain programs that included physical therapy, psychological interventions, and other non-medical treatments reported greater improvements in pain and quality of life compared to those who relied solely on medication or other medical treatments. (https://theacpa.org/multi-disciplinary-pain-programs/).

While these studies suggest that a comprehensive approach to managing chronic pain produces better outcomes than relying solely on medication or interventional procedures, it's essential to recognize that each person's experience with chronic pain is unique and necessitates an individualized SHRP approach.

It is also noteworthy to recognize that solely adhering to the medical model entails a significant human and financial cost. At the time of this publication, a recent estimated total economic burden of prescription opioid misuse in the United States was not available. However, the Centers for Disease Control and Prevention (CDC) estimated that the total economic burden of prescription opioid misuse in the United States in 2013 was $78.5 billion.[14]

Relying on pills to treat chronic pain might seem like the easy way out, but let's not forget the harsh reality of the situation. The undeniable truth is that the high risk of opioid dependence and overdose, including possible addiction, has become a massive public health crisis with plenty of blame to go around.

However, the impact of opioid abuse is not limited to individual health consequences. The economic burden of healthcare expenses, lost productivity, and criminal justice costs associated with opioid abuse is significant. This raises a critical question: Is the ease and convenience of relying on opioid medication and injections truly worth the overwhelming financial and human costs?

> ***This author overwhelmingly says, "No!"***

Dependence on pharmacological interventions for the management of chronic pain has given rise to unfavorable outcomes and complications, including but not limited to drowsiness, nausea, constipation, respiratory depression, cognitive impairment, mental health issues, and even death.

Apart from the human health and economic expenses, depending entirely on the medical model for pain management can also result in social costs. People may isolate themselves and refrain from participating in social activities and physical therapy, which can cause depression, anxiety, and a decreased quality of life.

In essence, the medical model is counterproductive as it can easily add to the "wind-up effect" discussed previously, causing the patient to feel more tense and potentially increasing or prolonging their experience of pain, in other words, amplifying their brain's sense of danger (a chronic pain cycle).

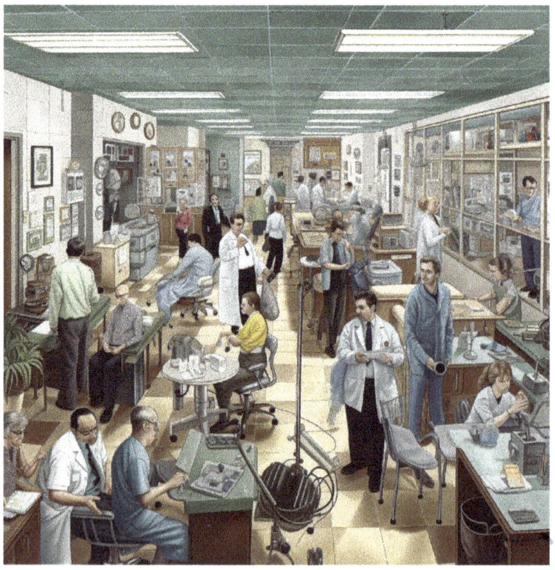

To reduce the risk of this pain amplification or sensitization of the nervous system and minimize the adverse effects associated with medication-based treatments, healthcare professionals, particularly physicians, must adopt a systematic approach to pain management. This involves incorporating non-pharmacological interventions that address the physical, psychological, and social aspects of chronic pain.

By adopting such an approach, physicians can help to reduce the nervous system's sensitization, improve patient outcomes, and increase adherence to treatment plans.

Several initiatives have recently been launched in response to the need for physicians to obtain resources and training in non-pharmacological pain management.

To close the gap in non-pharmacological pain management, healthcare providers need better training opportunities. As of November 2022, the CDC's website reported,

"Pain management is a significant public health issue that affects millions of Americans daily. In response, the CDC has released an updated set of clinical recommendations for healthcare providers who care for adult patients with short- and long-term pain."

These recommendations, outlined in the CDC Clinical Practice Guideline for Prescribing Opioids for Pain, prioritize safe and effective pain care, with a strong emphasis on non-pharmacological interventions such as physical therapy and behavioral health. This updated guideline in 2020 replaced the CDC's previous guideline for prescribing opioids for chronic pain, which was released in 2016.

The CDC has also created an online training program to help healthcare providers learn about non-pharmacological approaches to pain management[15]

Medical schools and residency programs are also stepping up to provide more training in non-pharmacological pain management. A survey by the Association of American Medical Colleges revealed that almost all participating schools included some pain management education in their curriculum, and many have increased training in non-pharmacological approaches.[16]

Another initiative is to increase access to non-pharmacological pain management resources for healthcare providers. The Veterans Health Administration (VHA) has implemented a national pain management strategy that includes establishing pain management teams, utilizing complementary and alternative medicine, and using telehealth to expand access to pain management resources.[17]

Advocacy for changes to insurance coverage policies is also gaining momentum to expand access to non-pharmacological pain management approaches. The American Physical Therapy Association is pushing to include physical therapy in Medicare and private insurance coverage for pain management.[18]

Overall, several ongoing initiatives address the lack of training and resources in non-pharmacological pain management approaches for physicians. These efforts aim to improve pain management outcomes and reduce reliance on pharmacological interventions for chronic pain.

Quotes To Spark
Thought And Discussion

"We have to change the way we think about addiction. We have to treat it as a health issue, not a criminal justice issue."

-Senator Chris Murphy

"The opioid epidemic is the biggest public health crisis facing America."

-Dr. Sanjay Gupta, CNN Chief Medical Correspondent

"The opioid epidemic is a symptom of a deeper problem in American society, and that problem is the dislocation and disconnection of individuals."

-Johann Hari, Author "Chasing the Scream: The First and Last Days of the War on Drugs."

“The greatest tragedy in life is the pain we suffer and the pain we miss. The moments of joy and connection that we forgo in our efforts to avoid discomfort.”

-Brené Brown, a research professor

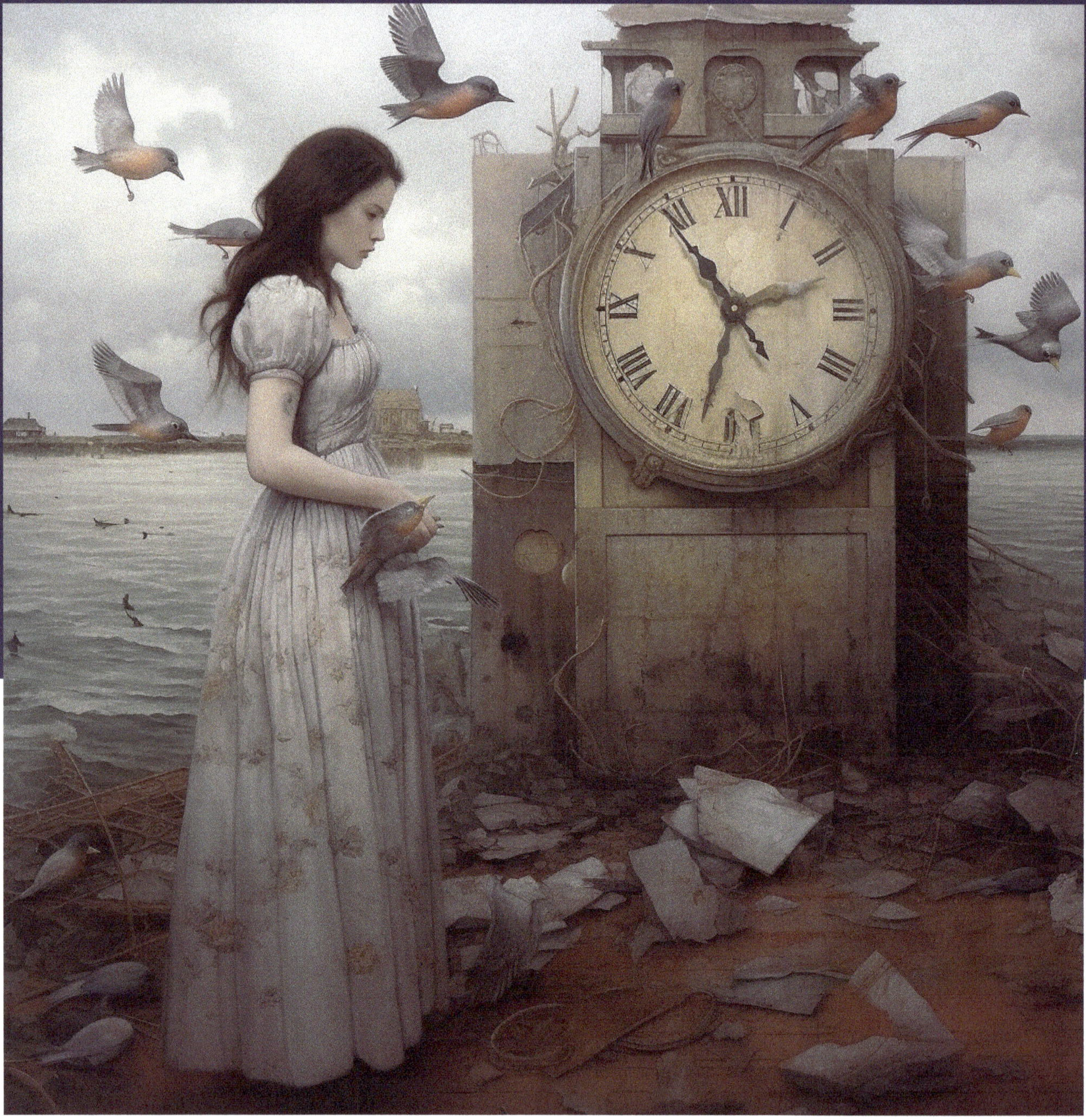

Chapter Four

Too Little...Too Late.

A true story...

"John had been living with chronic pain for 14 years. He had tried everything from physical therapy to acupuncture to manage his pain, but nothing seemed to work. Finally, his doctor recommended he try opioid therapy to help him manage his pain. At first, John was hesitant. He had heard all the stories about people becoming addicted to opioids and he didn't want to go down that path. But he was also desperate for relief from his pain, so he decided to give it a try.

At first, the opioids seemed to help. John was finally able to get some relief from his pain and start living his life again. But soon, he noticed the stigma that came with taking opioids. People would judge him when they found out he was taking them, assuming he was an addict looking for a fix, and they would say, "It's all in your head." John's doctor became skeptical of his opioid use. It made John feel like he was doing something wrong, even though he was trying to manage his chronic pain. Eventually, John decided to stop taking the opioids altogether.

He couldn't handle the stigma and judgment that came with them, even though they were the only thing that had provided him with some relief from his pain. He continued to live with chronic pain, feeling frustrated and misunderstood by the medical community."

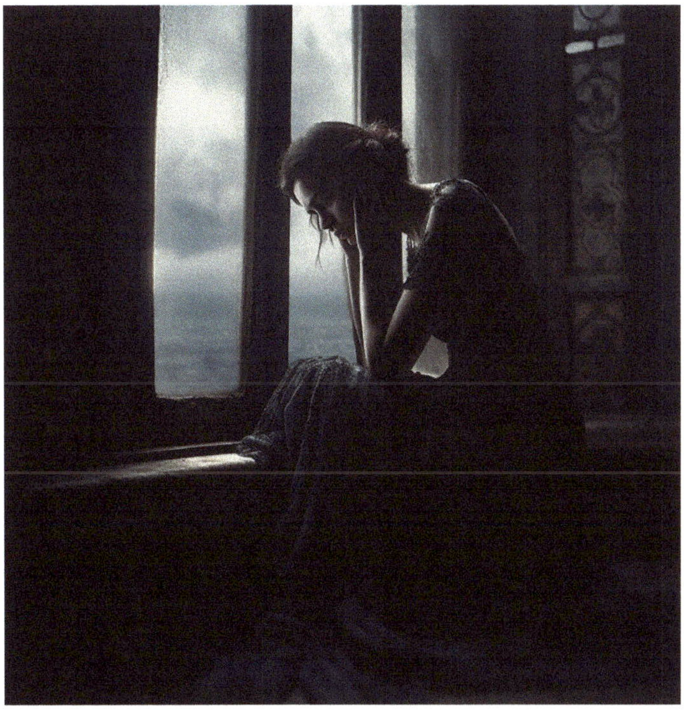

Could it be that John's pain has progressed to a point where it's too late to find relief? Additionally, what about the persistent obstacles that physicians face in implementing non-pharmacological approaches to pain management, such as limited training, insufficient resources, and personal biases? Is it too late?

While the answer to these questions may not be clear, what is certain is the toll that chronic pain can take on an individual. Chronic pain can be an overwhelming experience that significantly impacts one's quality of life. However, it's important to recognize that there are a variety of options available for managing chronic pain, even in seemingly hopeless cases.

Chronic pain can be a challenging and overwhelming experience that can interfere with one's quality of life. However, it's important to remember that various options for managing chronic pain are available, even if it seems too late.

As the above quote stated, "The greatest tragedy in life is the pain we suffer and the pain we miss...the moments of joy and connection that we forgo in our efforts to avoid discomfort." It's necessary to explore all possible approaches to pain management to achieve a more fulfilling life.

Thankfully, ongoing initiatives are being implemented to address the barriers that prevent physicians from utilizing non-pharmacological pain management approaches, such as inadequate training or resources, restricted insurance coverage, cultural prejudices, and personal beliefs and practices. By raising awareness and promoting education, we can work towards a better understanding of chronic pain and effective pain management.

To address inadequate training or resources, the Centers for Disease Control and Prevention (CDC) has developed an online training series called "The CDC Guideline for Prescribing Opioids for Chronic Pain," which aims to provide physicians with the necessary knowledge and skills to manage chronic pain safely and effectively.[19]

The training series includes modules on topics such as patient assessment, non-opioid treatments for chronic pain, opioid selection, and dosage, and patient follow-up and discontinuation.

In addition to the online training series, the CDC has also established the Prescription Drug Overdose: Prevention for States program, which provides funding and technical assistance to states to help them develop and implement strategies to prevent prescription drug overdose, including improving prescription drug monitoring programs, increasing access to naloxone, and enhancing pain management practices.[20]

Furthermore, the CDC is working to increase public awareness and education about chronic pain and its management through its "Know Your Pain" campaign, which includes resources and information for patients and healthcare providers. Overall, the CDC is taking a multifaceted approach to address the lack of adequate training and resources for physicians on chronic pain management.[21]

To address the lack of insurance coverage, advocacy efforts are being made to change insurance policies to increase access to non-pharmacological pain management approaches. The American Physical Therapy Association advocates including physical therapy in Medicare treatments and private insurance coverage for pain management.[22]

To address cultural bias, healthcare organizations are developing culturally sensitive approaches to pain management. For example, the National Institutes of Health's National Center for Complementary and Integrative Health funds research on using complementary and alternative medicine for pain management in diverse populations.[23]

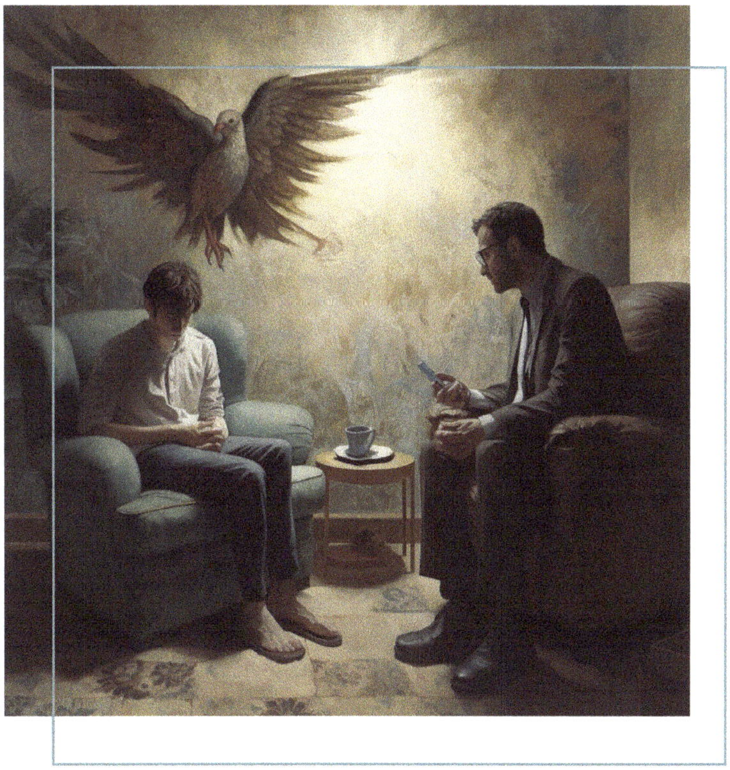

Finally, addressing personal beliefs and practices, efforts are being made to improve physician education on the risks and benefits of different pain management approaches. The CDC's guidelines for opioid prescribing emphasize the importance of informed decision-making and shared decision-making between patients and providers.[24]

These initiatives improve pain management outcomes and reduce the reliance on pharmacological interventions for chronic pain by addressing the various barriers to non-pharmacological approaches.

There are various reasons why current chronic pain management strategies may fall short of achieving their intended outcomes.

- ***Firstly,*** people may not fully engage in a treatment process or fail to recognize the benefits of non-pharmacological interventions, leading to non-compliance.
- **Secondly,** limited access to non-pharmacological interventions due to inadequate resources or insufficient insurance coverage may undermine the effectiveness of treatment.

- **Thirdly,** the lack of adequate training or knowledge in non-pharmacological modalities, such as neuropsychological education, the BPSS approach, and trauma-informed care, among physicians poses a significant challenge to the success of chronic pain treatment.
- **Fourthly,** cultural biases, personal beliefs, and current traditional practices may also hinder the effectiveness of treatment.
- **Finally,** a lack of interdisciplinary collaboration among healthcare providers hinders the integration of non-pharmacological interventions into a patient's treatment or care plan.

To achieve its goals, chronic pain treatment needs to recognize the intricate nature of chronic pain and incorporate evidence-based techniques, such as the Strategic Harm Reduction Plan. To effectively implement this model, one must possess a deep understanding of the intricate factors that shape the behavior of individuals with chronic pain.

To treat chronic pain effectively, including non-pharmacological evidence-based modalities in treatment plans is essential. SHRP is a prime example of an approach that integrates several modalities, including neuropsychological education, the Bio-Psycho-Social-Spiritual Pain (BPSS-P) approach, and trauma-informed care. This next quote sums up the nature's medical model:

> ***"The art of medicine consists of amusing the patient while nature cures the disease."***
>
> -Voltaire

The SHRP Approach emphasizes the power within individuals to improve their quality of life and manage their chronic pain through a combination of physical, psychological, and spiritual techniques.

Quotes To Spark
Thought And Discussion

"The reality of a chronic illness involves constant adjustments, struggles, and challenges. It's not just about living with pain, but also the social, emotional, and financial consequences that come with it."

-Donna L. Hamilton

"Living with chronic pain is like living with a wild animal. You never know when it will strike, how severe it will be, or how long it will last. It's always lurking in the shadows, waiting to pounce."

-John Durbin

"Chronic pain may be invisible, but it is a very real and all-consuming experience that affects every aspect of a person's life."

-Erica Stokes

"Living with chronic pain is like being in a never-ending battle with yourself. You want to do things, but your body won't let you. You want to be normal, but you're not."

-Glenn Banks

I can have less pain, more control, and a greater sense of safety. Prove it!"

-Chronic Pain Patient

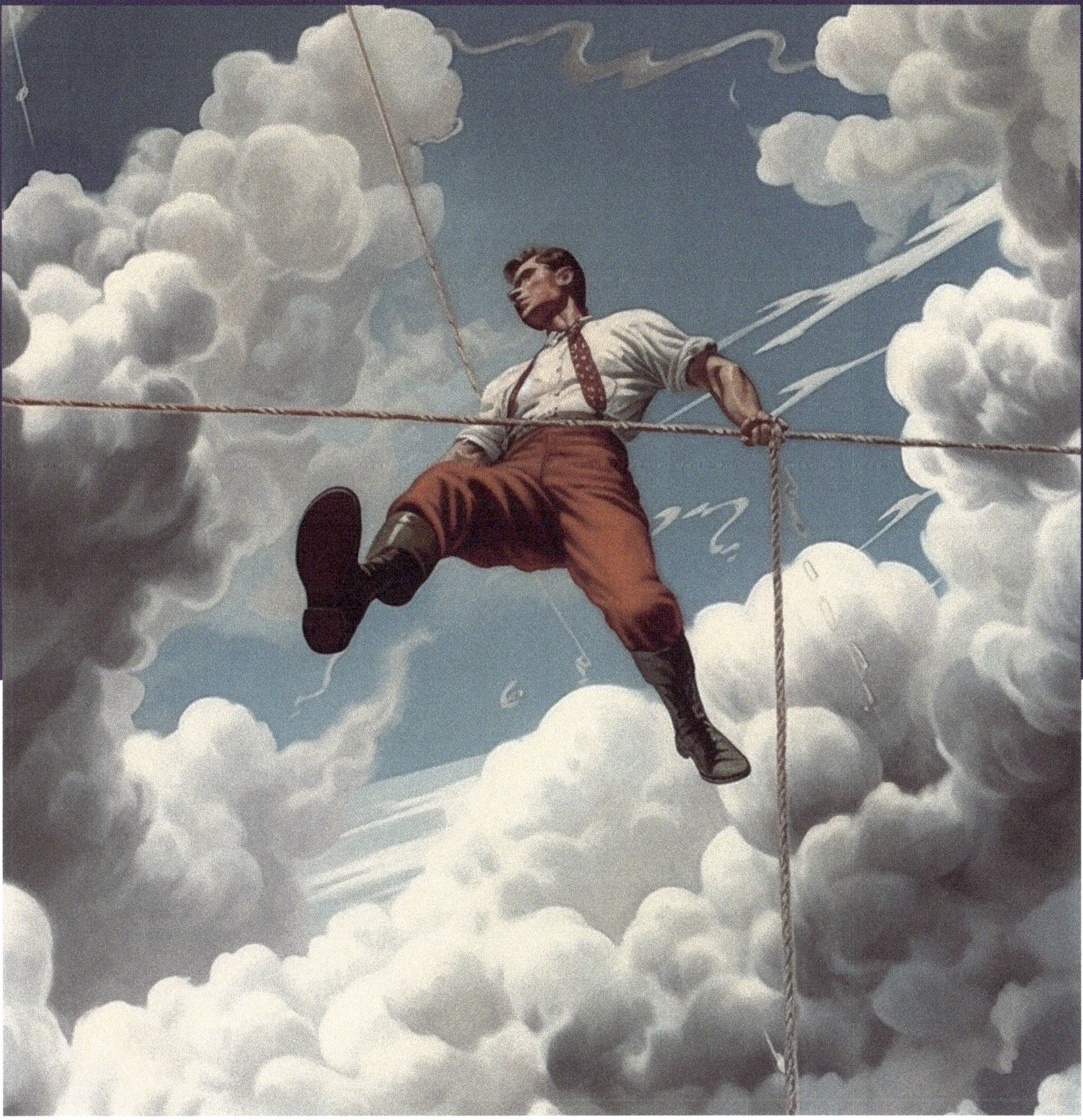

Chapter Five

The Pain Trifecta

To comprehensively address the complex nature of chronic pain, all chronic pain treatment needs to incorporate evidence-based practices, such as the SHRP approach.

This approach provides healthcare providers with thorough training and resources, overcomes financial barriers, confronts cultural biases and personal beliefs, and delves into the underlying psychological and emotional factors contributing to chronic pain.

To effectively address chronic pain, it's essential to prioritize improving overall functionality and well-being, rather than just symptom management. A patient-centered approach to chronic pain treatment, which is customized and thorough, can be highly effective in helping individuals manage their chronic pain and enhance their overall quality of life.

Neuro-Psych Education

The study of how the brain affects behavior and cognitive processes. It typically focuses on the relationships between brain structure and function, and how this affects mental processes such as attention, memory, language, and perception (Wind-up Effect; Safety).

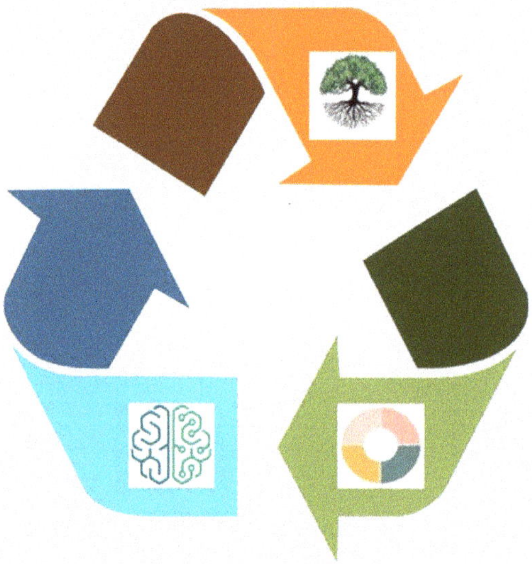

Trauma Informed Care

An approach that emphasizes understanding and responding to the impact of trauma on individuals in a compassionate and supportive way. The effects of trauma can be long-lasting and can influence an individual's ability to function in daily life, including their ability to form relationships, perform at work or school, and engage in self-care (1-5 patients; Pain seen as a threat).

BPSS Approach

The BPSS approach stands for Biological, Psychological, Social, and Spiritual, and is a framework used in healthcare and therapy to understand and address the various factors that contribute to an individual's overall health and well-being (Wind-down Areas).

Implementing the SHRP plan requires a deeper understanding of the intricate factors that shape the experiences and behavior of individuals with chronic pain. Success demands the integration of the three modalities, namely neuropsychological education, the Bio-Psycho-Social-Spiritual Pain (BPSS-P) approach, and trauma-informed care.

Neuropsychological Education

Neuropsychological education is a necessary first aspect of the SHRP plan, as it helps people comprehend the effects of their behavior on their brain and overall health. By educating patients about the connection between their actions and brain health, healthcare providers can empower them to participate actively in their care and improve adherence to treatment recommendations.

As a result, they are better equipped to make informed decisions and engage in behaviors that promote brain safety. Furthermore, incorporating neuropsychological education into a treatment plan can enhance patient-provider communication, leading to more personalized and effective treatment plans.

One study found that patients who received neuropsychological education were more likely to comply with treatment recommendations and had better outcomes than those who did not receive this education.[25]

The authors suggest that neuropsychological education may improve patient compliance by enhancing people's understanding of the consequences of their behavior and empowering them to take an active role in their care.

Educating people on the relationship between their behavior and the brain's sense of safety can aid in combating the stigma surrounding chronic pain. The emotional and behavioral changes that often accompany chronic pain can be difficult to handle and may worsen physical symptoms due to the "wind-up effect."

Unfortunately, the societal stigma surrounding chronic pain can make people feel isolated and ashamed, leading to further psychological distress and negative health outcomes, which increases central sensitization.

One study found that the stigma associated with chronic pain can lead to further psychological distress and negative health outcomes, which can increase central sensitization.[26]

Integrating neuropsychological education into compliance counseling can assist healthcare providers in conveying to patients that...

...chronic pain is not a personal failure or a reflection of their character.

People can gain insights that chronic pain can cause alterations in brain structure and function, which can affect behavior and mood. Such comprehension may contribute to reduced self-blame and shame, resulting in psychological well-being, improved pain management, and reduced wind-up effect.

Several studies have found that incorporating neuropsychological education into chronic pain management can result in improved psychological well-being and pain management.

For example, a randomized controlled trial found that patients who received neuropsychological education had significant improvements in pain, disability, and psychological functioning compared to a control group.[27]

Another study found that patients who received neuropsychological education had higher levels of self-efficacy and lower levels of pain catastrophizing compared to a control group.[28]

Furthermore, by educating patients on the relationship between behavior and the brain's sense of safety, providers can help them develop strategies to manage their pain better. Patients can learn techniques to manage stress, improve sleep, engage in physical activity, and develop healthy coping mechanisms.

As patients become more informed and empowered, they can gradually take an active role in their care and advocate for themselves, reducing the impact of chronic pain on their overall health and quality of life.

Bio-Psycho-Social-Spiritual Pain Approach

The BPSS-P approach is a necessary component of the SHRP plan, which aims to consider various factors that impact brain health and safety.

The model emphasizes the significance of addressing the underlying beliefs, preferences, and values that may influence patient behavior, allowing healthcare providers to develop personalized treatment plans that are more effective and acceptable to patients.[29]

While the model is relatively new, research has shown its effectiveness in addressing mental health issues such as anxiety and depression. Many articles emphasize the importance of the BPSS-P approach in promoting comprehensive healthcare, including chronic pain.[30]

One study found that the BPSS-P approach effectively improved treatment recommendations among patients with chronic pain. The authors suggest that the BPSS-P approach may be useful for patients with complex medical conditions like chronic pain, as it can help healthcare providers develop treatment plans meeting their unique needs and preferences.[31]

Trauma-Informed Care

Trauma-informed care (TIC) is an approach that acknowledges the prevalence and impact of trauma on patients' physical and mental health and emphasizes creating a safe and supportive environment for patients.

It is an important component of the SHRP plan, as studies have found that a significant portion of chronic pain patients have experienced trauma.

- For instance, Asmundson et al. (2004) found that 43% of patients seeking treatment for chronic pain reported a history of trauma, with 20% experiencing symptoms consistent with PTSD.[32]
- Similarly, Heinberg et al. (2006) found that 33% of chronic pain patients had a history of childhood abuse, which was associated with more severe pain and psychological distress.[33]
- Tietjen et al. (2015) estimated that 25-50% of chronic pain patients have a history of trauma, which is associated with worse pain outcomes and increased disability.[34]

(It's important to note that different studies use different definitions and measures of trauma, which can affect reported percentages).

Furthermore, trauma-informed care has been shown to improve adherence to treatment recommendations among patients with substance use disorders.[35]

Healthcare providers can use this approach to address underlying factors that may contribute to non-adherence, particularly among patients with co-occurring mental health conditions or a history of trauma.

Quotes To Spark Thought And Discussion

"There is hope, even when your brain tells you there isn't."

-John Green

"Pain is inevitable, but suffering is optional. We cannot avoid pain, but we can avoid the suffering caused by the pain."

-Buddha

"The goal of chronic pain management isn't to eliminate pain, but to reduce it to a manageable level and improve quality of life."

-Glenn Banks

"Your brain's number one job is not to think or feel, but to keep you alive and safe. Everything it does, including thinking and feeling, serves that primary purpose."

-Rick Hanson, senior fellow of the Greater Good Science Center at UC Berkeley

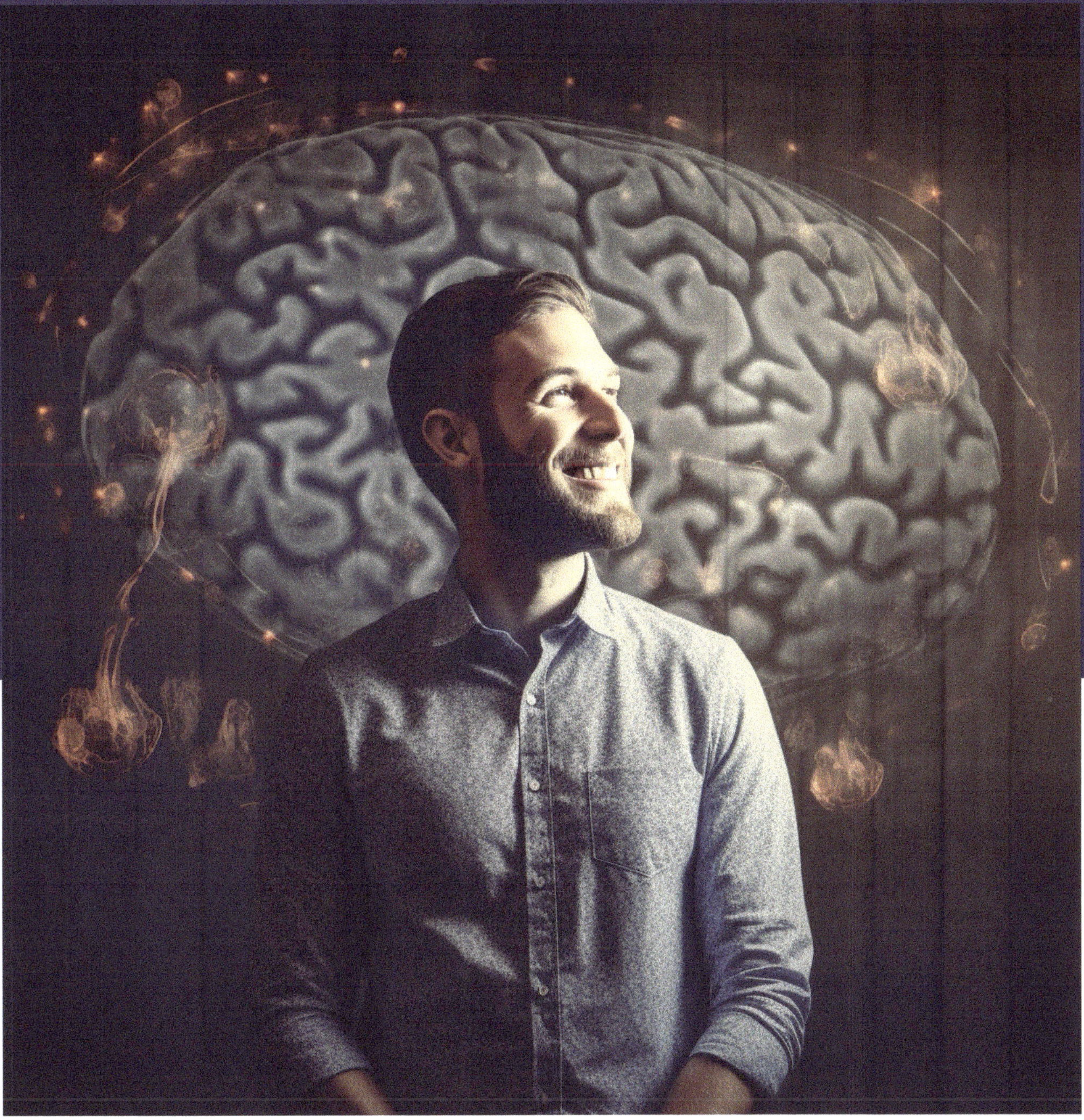

Chapter Six

Embrace Safety

The brain's response to a perceived threat is important for creating a sense of safety because it influences an individual's thoughts, emotions, and behaviors. For example, if an individual has experienced trauma in the past, their brain may be more sensitive to potential threats in the environment, which can lead to increased anxiety, hyper-vigilance, and avoidance behaviors. In contrast, if an individual has experienced positive experiences, their brain may be more attuned to positive aspects of the environment, leading to feelings of safety and security.

As per the ***Central Sensitization Theory*** [36], chronic pain is perceived as a threat by the brain after an average of six to eight months of continuous pain signaling to the brain, like the bear in the woods discussed in Chapter Two. This is because the nervous system becomes progressively more sensitive and responsive to various stimuli, including pain signals.

Central Sensitization is a phenomenon in which the brain "learns" to interpret pain as a greater threat, leading to an increased sensitivity response that results in stable or increased pain. The brain does its job by alerting us to a continued threat.

However, since the pain persists, the brain reduces the threat by increasing our sensitivity. It's important to recognize this process and seek appropriate treatment to address the underlying medical and psychological cause of the pain, rather than just managing the symptoms.

Chronic pain is a complex condition that is influenced by a variety of factors, including biological, psychological, and social components. It is thought that chronic pain can result from changes in the neurotransmitters and receptors involved in pain processing, as well as alterations in the structure and function of the brain's neural circuits.[37][38] These changes can cause chronic pain to become self-sustaining, even in the absence of ongoing tissue damage or injury.[39]

In many cases, chronic pain can trigger the wind-up effect, a phenomenon, as stated before, in which pain signals become amplified and persistent, leading to a cycle of increasing pain and sensitivity.[40]

Chronic pain can become a significant threat to individuals as it triggers pain pathways in the brain, creating a continuous loop even in the absence of actual tissue damage or injury. This phenomenon, known as the wind-up effect, presents a significant obstacle to finding relief through conventional pain management approaches, including medication and physical therapy.[41]

Given this reality, knowing how individuals mitigate chronic pain is like the bear in the woods (a threat). Remember the story of Judy walking in the woods?

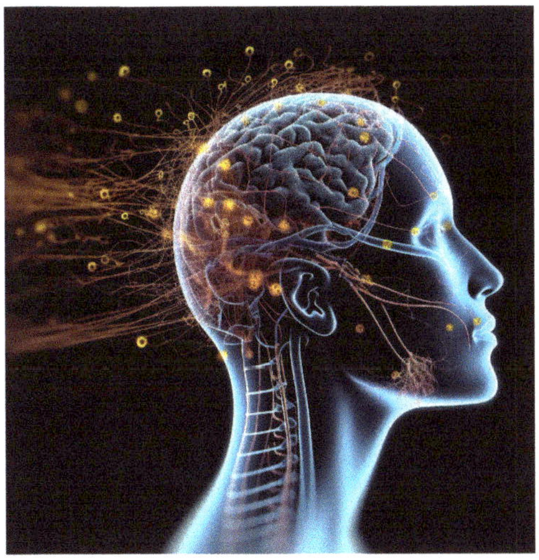

"Judy has developed a keen sense of hyper-vigilance during her daily hikes in the woods, convinced that a bear may lurk nearby despite never having encountered one. Although she has never faced any immediate danger, her persistent state of anxiety keeps her constantly on edge, ensuring that she remains in a state of heightened alertness."

Therefore, it is imperative to address chronic pain using a multifaceted approach that considers the biological, psychological, and social components of the condition. This approach may include non-pharmacological pain management techniques, such as cognitive-behavioral therapy, mindfulness-based stress reduction, and physical therapy.

Additionally, it may involve medication-assisted treatment, which combines medication with behavioral therapies to address both the physical and psychological aspects of chronic pain.[42]

Chronic pain is a condition that can be difficult to treat using traditional pain management approaches. Understanding the mechanisms behind chronic pain and the wind-up effect can help healthcare providers develop more effective strategies to manage chronic pain and improve the overall quality of life for individuals experiencing chronic pain.

There are additional resources on chronic pain being seen as a threat and have contributed greatly to developing the Strategic Harm Reduction Plan. The above studies demonstrate that chronic pain can alter the brain's structure and function, leading to increased sensory processing, emotional regulation, and cognitive function.[43abcd] The scientific definition of this is called Neuroplasticity.

Quotes To Spark
Thought And Discussion

"Chronic pain is not the same as acute pain. Acute pain is a normal sensation triggered in the nervous system to alert you to possible injury and the need to take care of yourself. Chronic pain persists. Pain signals keep firing in the nervous system for weeks, months, even years."

-American Chronic Pain Association

"Chronic pain is a condition that is very different from acute pain. While acute pain is a normal sensation that alerts us to possible injury, chronic pain persists long after the injury has healed."

-National Institute of Neurological Disorders and Stroke

"Acute pain is a symptom of injured or diseased tissue. Chronic pain, on the other hand, is a condition in its own right."

-British Pain Society

"You might not be able to teach an old dog new tricks, but you sure can give him or her new toys to play with."

-Glenn Banks

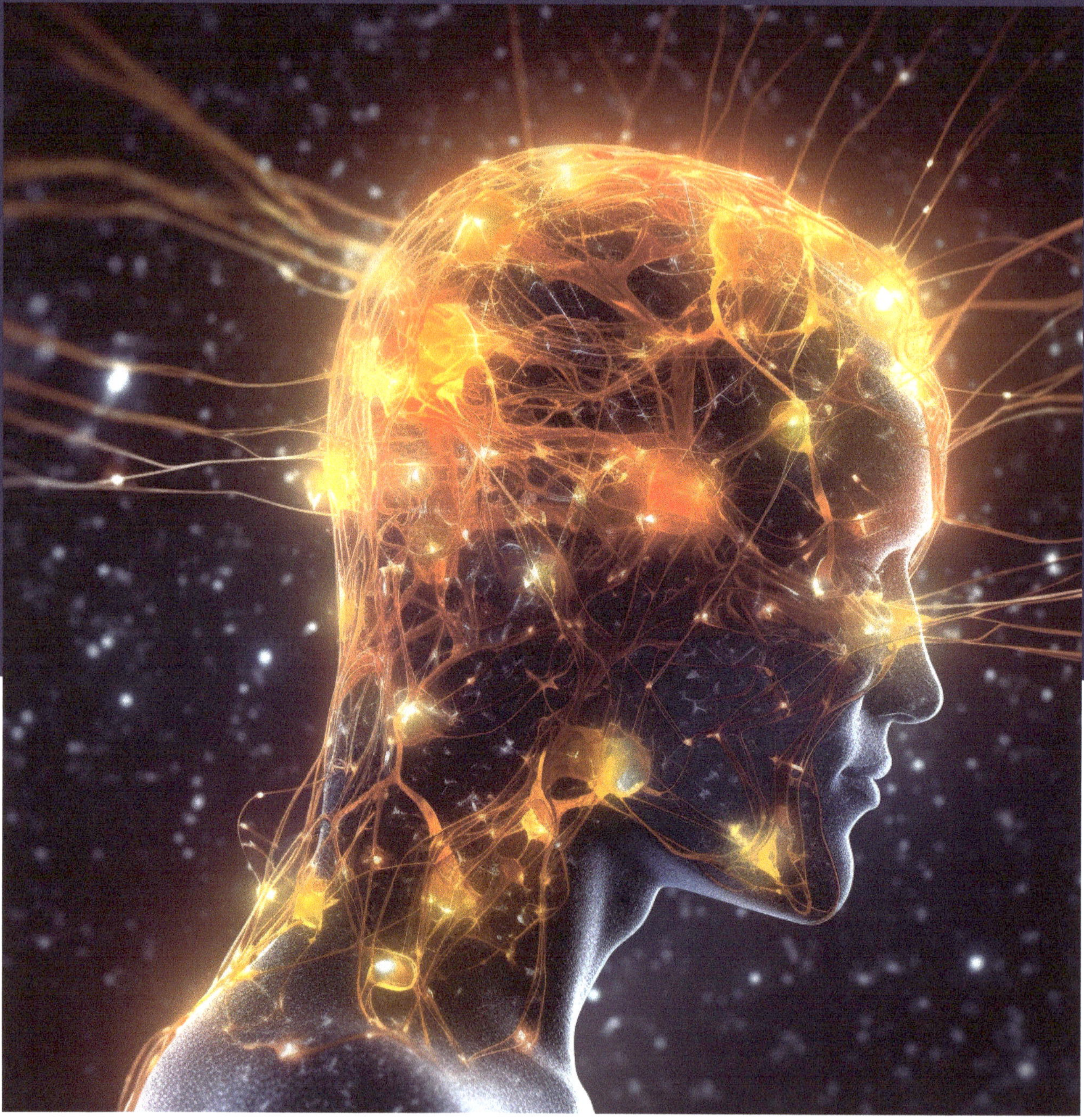

Chapter Seven

Harnessing Neuroplasticity

Age does not dictate one's ability to learn new skills. With commitment, time, and effort, it's possible to teach old dogs new tricks. Neuroplasticity is the brain's capability to physically change its structure and adapt to different experiences, behaviors, and environmental factors, vital for learning, memory, and recovery from neurological disorders or injuries.

Recent research has focused on utilizing neuroplasticity to improve cognitive and motor functions in various populations, including individuals with Parkinson's disease, stroke patients, and aging adults.

Different interventions, such as physical exercise, cognitive training, and non-invasive brain stimulation, have been studied to determine their effectiveness in promoting neuroplasticity and enhancing brain function.

An inspiring story...

"A person who was able to change his habits through neuroplasticity is Michael Merzenich, a renowned neuroscientist. In his 60s, he realized that he was beginning to experience some cognitive decline and decided to take matters into his own hands by developing a brain training program.

Merzenich spent years studying the principles of neuroplasticity and applied them to create a set of exercises aimed at improving cognitive function. He practiced these exercises for hours every day and over time, he saw significant improvements in his memory, attention, and overall mental clarity.

Not only did Merzenich's program benefit himself, but it also helped thousands of others who used his methods to improve their brain function."

Michael's story is a powerful example of how perseverance and a commitment to increasing targeted neuroplasticity can lead to actual structural changes in the brain, even later in life.

Neuroplasticity enables the brain to adapt and restructure itself in response to various experiences and environmental factors, including prolonged chronic pain.

"Neuroplasticity allows the brain to rewrite its software, allowing us to change the way we think and behave."

-Dr. Norman Doidge, a psychiatrist and psychoanalyst

This adaptability can lead to physical changes in the brain's structure that also may be maladaptive, resulting in altered pain signal processing, increased pain sensitivity, and changes in mood, cognition, and behavior.[44]

In other words, chronic pain can cause the brain to rewire itself, potentially exacerbating the experience of pain and its associated effects on mental health and daily functioning.[45] Recent studies have investigated the use of neuroplasticity-based interventions to treat chronic pain.

For example, a study published in the Journal of Pain (2021) demonstrated that High-Definition transcranial Direct Current Stimulation (HD-tDCS), a neuroplasticity-based intervention, significantly improved pain and function in individuals with chronic knee osteoarthritis.[46]

Similarly, a study published in Brain in 2020 showed that a mindfulness-based intervention improved neuroplasticity and reduced pain in individuals with chronic low back pain.[47]

Before we go on...let's recap what we have learned so far!

After approximately six to eight months of experiencing daily chronic pain signaling, the brain has the potential to perceive the pain itself as a threat due to central sensitization. This physical change in the brain occurs when the brain's response to pain signals becomes increasingly amplified over time, exacerbating the experience of chronic pain. Despite adhering to prescribed treatment requirements, individuals struggle to manage their chronic pain effectively.

"Neurons that fire together, wire together."

-Donald Hebb

Chronic pain changes the brain's physical structure and function, abnormally increasing sensory processing, emotional regulation, and cognitive function. These changes contribute to the development of co-morbid conditions, such as depression, anxiety, and sleep disturbances.

Therefore, early intervention is needed to prevent the "wind-up effect" from occurring, after central sensitization, and avoid potential long-term neurological consequences. In cases where the effect has already happened, the SHRP plan will induce a wind-down effect through neuroplasticity, ultimately providing relief and improving overall well-being.

Quotes To Spark
Thought And Discussion

"Neuroplasticity is the brain's ability to reorganize itself by forming new neural connections throughout life. It is real and why rehabilitation after injury or stroke is possible."

-Dr. Michael Merzenich, neuroscientist and co-founder of Posit Science.

"Neuroplasticity is not fiction, but instead the marvelous reality of our brains' ability to change and adapt."

-Dr. Norman Doidge, psychiatrist and author of "The Brain That Changes Itself".

"Neuroplasticity is a real phenomenon. The human brain is remarkably adaptable and constantly changes in response to new experiences, learning, and recovery from injury."

-Dr. Alvaro Pascual-Leone, neurologist and director of the Berenson-Allen Center for Noninvasive Brain Stimulation at Harvard Medical School.

Quotes To Spark
Thought And Discussion

"The brain's ability to change and adapt is one of the most remarkable discoveries of the last century. This phenomenon, known as neuroplasticity, is real, and holds the promise of healing and recovery for millions of people."

-Dr. Sharon Begley, author of "Train Your Mind, Change Your Brain".

"The idea that the brain is fixed and unchangeable is outdated. We now know that the brain is constantly changing, adapting, and evolving, a process known as neuroplasticity."

-Dr. Daniel J. Siegel, Professor of Psychiatry - UCLA, author of "The Mindful Brain".

"All for one and one for all, united we stand divided we fall."

-Alexandre Dumas

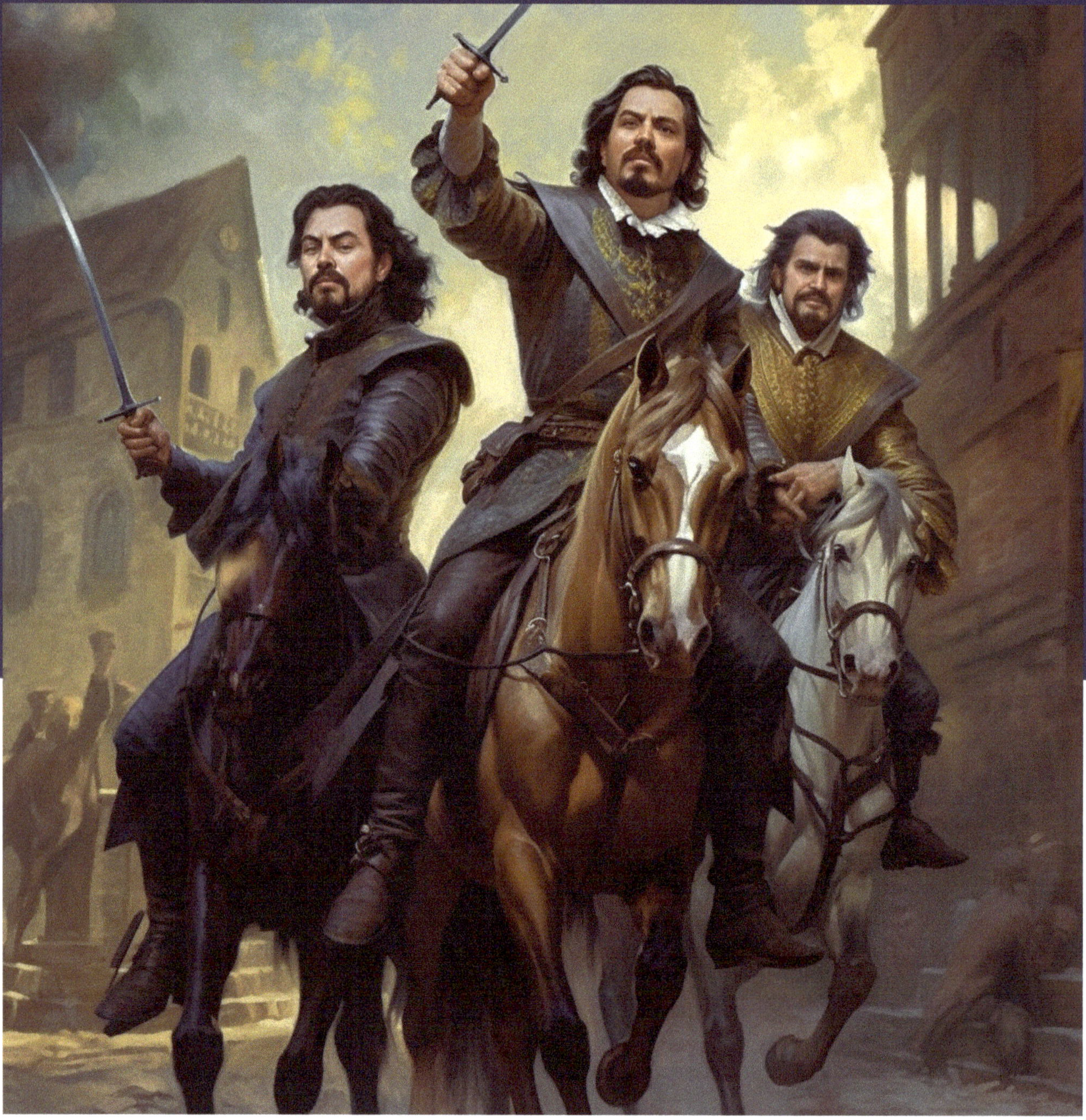

Chapter Eight

Prioritizing Brain Health

The famous motto "All for one and one for all" originated from Alexandre Dumas' novel "The Three Musketeers". The phrase symbolizes the unwavering loyalty and commitment of the musketeers to work together as a team to overcome obstacles, highlighting the importance of unity and support during challenging times.

In the context of the SHRP plan, the three musketeers are represented by Athos, who stands for neuropsychological education, Porthos, who represents the BPSS approach, and D'Artagnan, who embodies trauma-informed care.

These three areas of study are essential factors that significantly impact brain safety, and when combined, they play a pivotal role in promoting brain safety and improving overall brain health.

Brain safety is a concept that encompasses various measures and practices that are implemented to promote and maintain the health and well-being of the brain. It involves a wide range of factors that can impact the function and structure of the brain, such as protecting against injury, managing stress, maintaining a healthy lifestyle, and preventing or treating conditions like chronic pain.

It's quite ironic that even though the brain is arguably the most important organ in our body, most people fail to prioritize brain health and safety. Taking care of our brain is vital since it controls various aspects of our physical, cognitive, and emotional functioning. Despite this, some individuals seem to neglect the importance of brain safety, even though it's essential for people of all ages and backgrounds.

To promote brain safety and ensure optimal brain health, it is important to start by educating ourselves on the brain's structure, function, and vulnerability. This educational process should include a thorough understanding of the various factors that can impact brain health, including injury, stress, lifestyle choices, and mental health conditions. Remember…

"The pain is not in your head, but the solution is not in your body!"

By increasing our awareness of the brain's vulnerability, we can take appropriate measures to protect it, such as adopting healthy habits, managing stress, and seeking better medical care when necessary.

As a result, education and awareness play a vital role in promoting brain safety. To this end, the SHRP plan emphasizes patient education as the first step toward optimal brain health.

By providing patients with a comprehensive understanding of their brain safety measures, the SHRP plan empowers individuals to control their brain health, make informed decisions that support their overall well-being, and begin to control the wind-up effect.

The metaphorical representation of the three musketeers underscores the significance of these three areas collaborating in harmony towards a common objective.

Let's dig deeper into the word "safety", because nothing screams safety quite like challenging our brain's capacity to feel safe.

When a person says that he or she is safe, it typically means that the person feels protected from harm or danger. This feeling of safety can be both physical and emotional. In a physical sense, safety can refer to being protected from injury, or physical danger. This may include feeling secure in one's surroundings, being free from physical threats or harm, or securing resources that provide physical safety, such as emergency services.

In an emotional sense, safety can refer to feeling secure and free from emotional harm or distress. This may include feeling comfortable and supported in one's relationships, having a sense of trust and safety in social situations, and feeling free from anxiety, fear, or trauma-related symptoms.

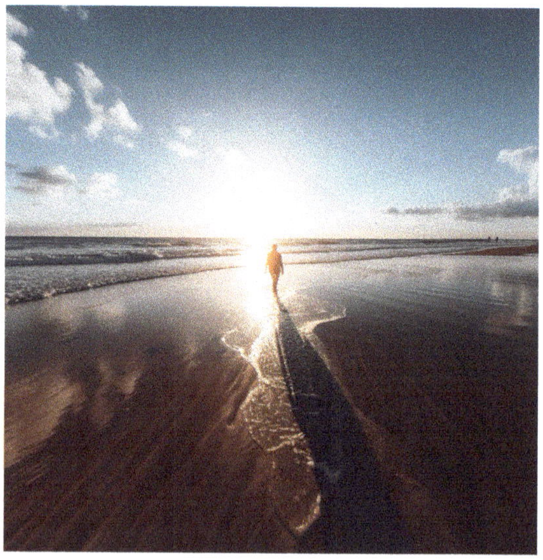

In general, the statement "I am safe" implies that the individual is experiencing a feeling of security and protection, which can encompass physical and emotional aspects, among others.

The SHRP plan incorporates several valuable modalities, including neuropsychological education, the BPSS approach, and trauma-informed care. However, brain safety is the overarching theme that unifies these three approaches.

It emphasizes the importance of healthcare providers prioritizing safe interventions and minimizing the risk of harm to the patient's sense of safety while avoiding any exacerbation of the "wind-up effect".

In the context of the SHRP plan, brain safety becomes important as patients, and others in their sphere of influence may be vulnerable to harm resulting from non-adherence to treatment recommendations or the use of medications or treatments with potential side effects.

Ironic...nothing makes a person feel more safe and secure than his or her brain, which is constantly reminding them of all the things that could go wrong.

Prioritizing the brain's sensing safety is paramount and highlights the importance of utilizing non-pharmacological interventions whenever possible. These interventions, such as exercise, physical therapy, and mindfulness-based approaches, are safe, backed by evidence, and generally carry fewer potential side effects than medications. Healthcare providers can enhance the safety and well-being of their patients' brains and overall health by endorsing and supporting the implementation of these interventions, thereby reducing the risk of harm and fostering a greater sense of security.

Another important aspect of brain safety is monitoring patients for potential side effects of medications or treatments. This includes regularly assessing patients for signs of medication side effects, such as cognitive impairment or mood changes, and adjusting medications or dosages as needed to minimize the risk of harm.

In addition, healthcare providers should also consider the patient's overall health and well-being when making treatment recommendations. This includes considering the patient's medical history, current medications, and any underlying health conditions that may increase the risk of harm from certain treatments or medications.

Healthcare providers must prioritize creating a safe and supportive environment for individuals. A safe and secure healthcare environment involves not only the provision of quality care but also the physical surroundings of the healthcare facility.

An uncluttered and organized environment can contribute to patient safety and reduce the risk of errors or accidents.[48] Moreover, appropriate measures should be in place to prevent the spread of infections, such as proper hand hygiene practices and regular cleaning and disinfecting of high-touch surfaces.[49]

Additionally, healthcare facilities should provide adequate security measures to ensure the safety of patients, staff, and visitors.[50]

Furthermore, healthcare providers can create a safe and secure healthcare environment. They must prioritize patient safety, communicate effectively with patients and their families, and implement evidence-based practices to minimize the risk of errors or adverse events.[51]

Isn't it awesome to know that the brain is amazing at creating a sense of safety? After all, nothing says safety like activating the autonomic nervous system, releasing stress hormones, and altering cognitive and emotional processing in response to a perceived threat. Who needs a calm and rational response when you can have a full-blown fight-or-flight-or-freeze reaction right?

The brain plays an important role in ensuring a person's physical and psychological safety, as it serves as the primary regulator and coordinator of the body's responses.[52] It processes various stimuli, including those that may pose a threat or danger to the body.[53]

The brain continuously scans the environment for potential threats and triggers appropriate responses to safeguard the body from harm. These responses can be physical, such as fight-or-flight-or-freeze reactions, or cognitive and emotional, such as fear or anxiety.[54]. The brain's central role in promoting safety and survival is critical for overall well-being and optimal functioning.[55]

Here are other sources that discuss the central role of the brain in creating and maintaining safety:

- This book discusses the Polyvagal Theory, which proposes that the brain regulates autonomic responses to stress and threat. According to this theory, the brain's primary function is ***maintaining safety*** and regulating social engagement behaviors. Porges, S. W. (2011). The Polyvagal Theory: Neurophysiological Foundations of Emotions, Attachment, Communication, and Self-regulation. New York: W.W. Norton & Company.

- This book explores the impact of trauma on the brain and the body's responses to stress and threat. It highlights the central role of the brain in regulating responses to threats and emphasizes the importance of ***creating a sense of safety*** to facilitate healing from trauma. Van der Kolk, B. A. (2014). The Body Keeps the Score: Brain, Mind, and Body in the Healing of Trauma. New York: Penguin Books.
- This book discusses the brain's role in generating fear and anxiety responses and emphasizes the importance of understanding these responses to manage and treat anxiety-related disorders. It highlights the role of the brain in creating a sense of safety and reducing anxiety. Ledoux, J. (2015). Anxious: Using the Brain to Understand and Treat Fear and Anxiety. New York: Penguin Books.

The above sources emphasize the critical role of the brain in maintaining safety and regulating responses to stress and threat, indicating a sense of safety is imperative for promoting healing and well-being.

Therefore, healthcare providers must prioritize establishing safe and supportive environments for their patients to enhance patient safety and mitigate the risk of errors or adverse events.

Incorporating the techniques of the SHRP plan can contribute to creating a safe and supportive environment, promoting an increased sense of safety, and significantly reducing the wind-up effect for individuals with chronic pain.

While complete pain relief may be challenging, this approach helps wind down the wind-up effect, improve overall well-being, and provide greater control over chronic pain symptoms.

Thus, the Strategic Harm Reduction Plan offers individuals with chronic pain the opportunity to experience reduced pain, an increased sense of control, and enhanced feelings of safety and protection.

Quotes To Spark
Thought And Discussion

"Pain is not just a physical sensation. It is processed and modulated by the brain, which means that psychological factors, such as emotions, beliefs, and expectations, can influence the pain experience."

-Vania Apkarian, Professor of Physiology, Northwestern University

"Pain is not a single, monolithic entity. It is multidimensional and influenced by biological, psychological, and social factors. This means that effective pain management requires an integrated approach that addresses all aspects of the pain experience."

-Judith Turner, Prof of Psychiatry and Behavioral Sciences, Univ. of Wash.

"Chronic pain significantly impacts brain health, including cognitive function, mood, and quality of life. Managing chronic pain requires not just pain reduction, but also strategies to improve brain health and overall well-being."

-Heather Tick, Clinical Associate Professor, University of Washington

Quotes To Spark
Thought And Discussion

"Managing chronic pain is not just about treating the symptoms, but also about addressing the underlying factors that contribute to the pain experience, including brain function and emotional well-being."

-Beth Darnall, Clinical Professor, Stanford University

"Taking care of your brain is essential for managing chronic pain. This includes mindfulness, cognitive-behavioral therapy, and other mind-body techniques that can help regulate the nervous system and reduce pain."

-Robert Bonakdar, Director of Pain Management, Scripps Center for Integrative Medicine.

"Here we have a class of drugs that I can give you to relieve your pain,but they're also highly addictive, and if you take them for too long, they can make your pain worse. It's like a cruel joke."

-Dr. Travis Rieder, a bioethicist and author of the book, "In Pain: A Bioethicist's Personal Struggle with Opioids."

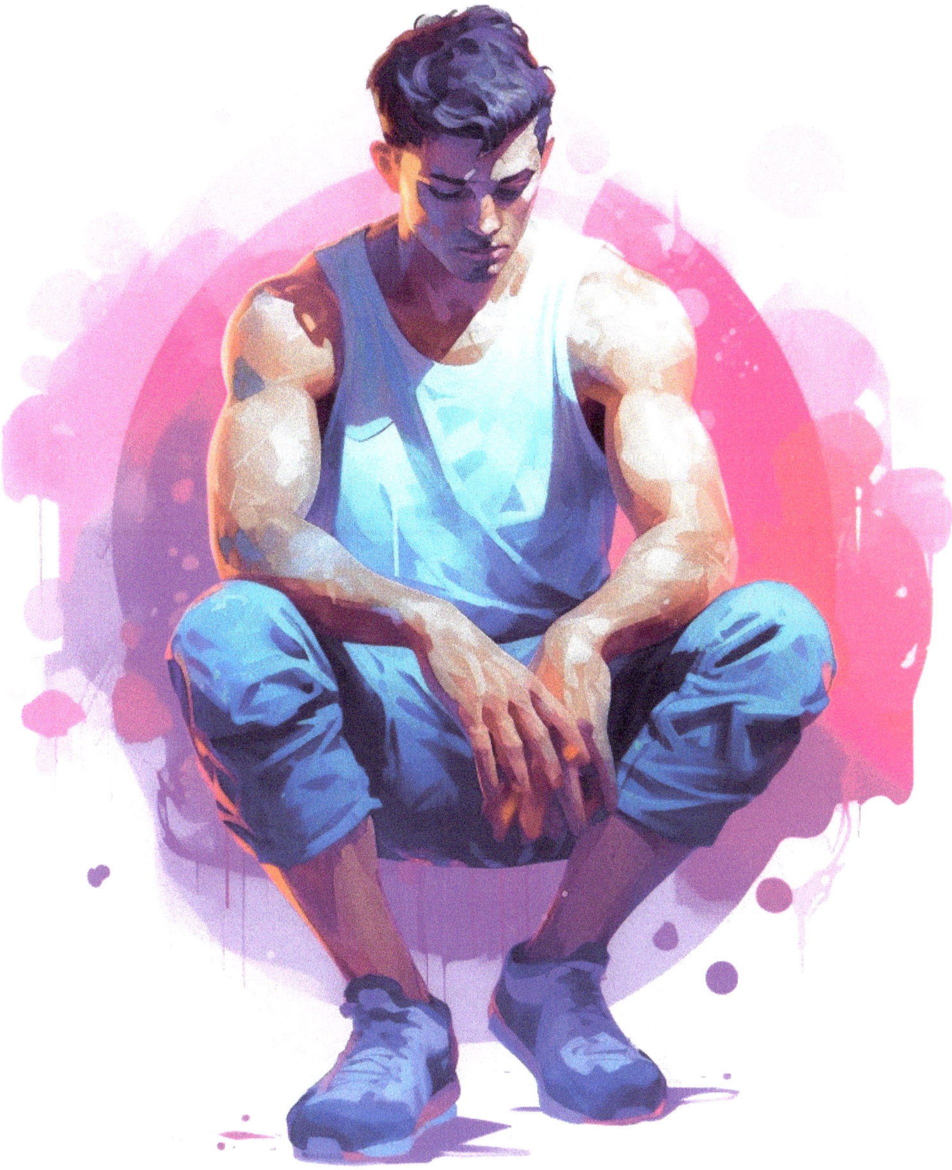

Chapter Nine

Opioid Irony

Chronic pain is a debilitating condition that affects millions of people worldwide. As stated, it can be caused by a variety of conditions such as arthritis, back pain, neuropathy, and cancer. For many years, opioid medication has been used to manage chronic pain due to its effectiveness in relieving pain. However, the overuse of opioid medication has become a significant public health concern.

The background of the overuse of opioid medication can be traced back to the late 1990s when pharmaceutical companies began aggressively marketing opioid medication as a safe and effective treatment for chronic pain. They claimed that opioid medication was not addictive, which led to doctors prescribing opioids more frequently to their patients.

As a result, the number of prescriptions for opioid medication increased significantly, leading to widespread misuse and abuse of these drugs. Many patients who were prescribed opioids for chronic pain became dependent and then addicted to the medication, leading to a rise in opioid-related deaths.

The significance of the overuse of opioid medication is that it has become a public health crisis. According to the Centers for Disease Control and Prevention (CDC), there were nearly 50,000 opioid-related overdose deaths in 2019 in the United States alone. The misuse and abuse of opioid medication have also led to an increase in hospital admissions, emergency room visits, and healthcare costs.

The overuse of opioid medication in combating chronic pain has become a significant public health concern due to its widespread misuse and abuse, leading to dependence, overdoses, and other serious health consequences. Healthcare providers must explore alternative treatments and manage the use of opioid medication more carefully to ensure that patients receive effective pain relief while avoiding the risks associated with opioid medication.

Opioids are a class of drugs that are primarily used to relieve pain. They work by binding to opioid receptors in the brain and spinal cord, reducing the perception of pain. While opioids have been effective in treating acute pain, such as pain from surgery or injury, their use for chronic pain management has been controversial.

In recent years, research has shown that opioids may not be effective in treating chronic pain and can lead to tolerance, dependence, possible addiction, overdose, and death. The following articles and studies suggest that opioids might not help chronic pain.

On April 5, 2023, NBC News published an article titled "Opioids are not the best medicine for chronic pain," reporting on a study published in the Journal of the American Medical Association. The study found that opioids were no more effective than non-opioid medications for managing chronic pain, and patients who took opioids were more likely to experience side effects such as constipation, nausea, and dizziness, among others.[56]

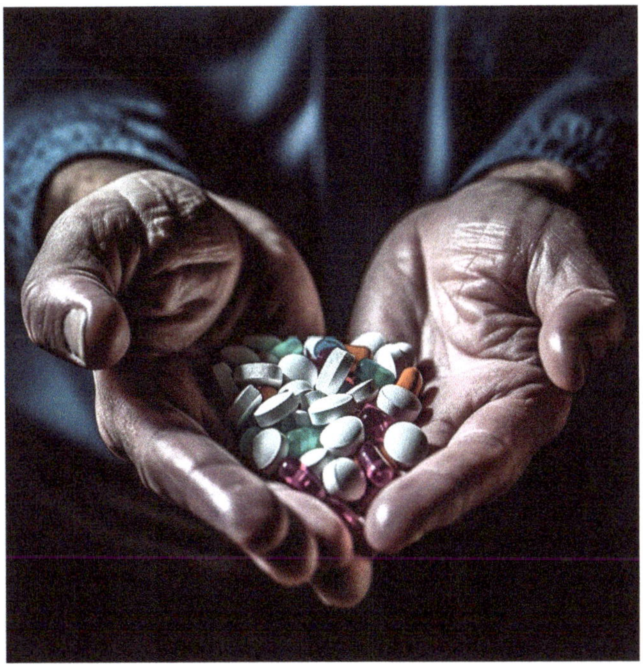

Similarly, the Harvard Health Blog article titled "Why opioids are not the best medicine for chronic pain" on March 22, 2023, discussed the risks and limitations of opioids for chronic pain management. The article highlighted alternative therapies such as physical therapy, cognitive-behavioral therapy, and non-opioid medications. The article noted that while opioids may provide short-term pain relief, they can also lead to dependence, possible addiction, overdose, and other serious complications.[57]

Furthermore, a systematic review of 62 randomized controlled trials summarized in the Medical News Today article titled "Opioids not effective for chronic pain, a new study confirms" on February 27, 2023, found that opioids were not effective for managing chronic pain. Like the other studies, the review found that opioids were associated with a higher risk of adverse effects compared to non-opioid medications, and alternative therapies should be considered for chronic pain management.[58]

As shown, there is a growing body of research indicating that opioids may not be the optimal approach for managing chronic pain. Although opioids have been successful in treating acute pain, their use for chronic pain management remains a contentious issue.

As highlighted in the studies, opioids have limited effectiveness in providing pain relief for chronic pain, and their use can result in harmful side effects. Therefore, there are several compelling reasons why opioids are proving to be an inadequate option for managing chronic pain in the long term.

- **Tolerance:** With long-term use, opioids can lead to tolerance, which means that the body becomes accustomed to the drug and requires higher doses to achieve the same level of pain relief. This can lead to a dangerous cycle of increasing doses and potential addiction.[59] According to the Centers for Disease Control and Prevention, over 81,000 drug overdose deaths occurred in the United States from May 2020 to May 2021, with synthetic opioids like fentanyl being the leading cause of overdose deaths.

- **Dependence and addiction:** Long-term use of opioids can also lead to dependence and addiction. Dependence occurs when the body becomes physically reliant on the drug and experiences withdrawal symptoms if it is stopped, or the dose is reduced. Addiction is a chronic disease characterized by compulsive drug seeking and use, despite harmful consequences.[60] The American Society of Addiction Medicine reports that 2 million people in the United States had a substance use disorder involving prescription opioids in 2018, and 130 people die every day from opioid-related drug overdoses.

- **Side effects:** Opioids can cause a range of side effects, including nausea, constipation, dizziness, confusion, and respiratory depression. These side effects can interfere with daily activities and reduce quality of life.[61] A study published in the Journal of Pain Research found that patients taking opioids for chronic pain developed tolerance to the drug over time, requiring higher doses for the same level of pain relief.

- **Overdose:** Opioids are associated with a high risk of overdose, which can lead to respiratory failure and death. In recent years, opioid overdose deaths have become a public health crisis in many countries.[62] The National Institute on Drug Abuse reports that common side effects of opioids include constipation, nausea, dizziness, and sedation. Long-term use can also cause hormonal imbalances, immune system suppression, and increased risk of falls and fractures.

- **Alternative treatments:** There are many alternative treatments available for chronic pain that do not carry the same risks as opioids, including physical therapy, cognitive-behavioral therapy, and non-opioid medications. These treatments can be just as effective for many patients with chronic pain.[63] A review of studies published in the Journal of the American Medical Association found that non-opioid treatments like physical therapy, cognitive behavioral therapy, and acupuncture were just as effective as opioids in managing chronic pain, with fewer side effects and lower risk of dependence and addiction.

Opioids are not the optimal option for managing chronic pain, despite their effectiveness in treating acute pain. Although they remain a topic of debate for long-term pain management, numerous studies have shown that opioids provide limited relief for chronic pain and can cause harmful side effects.

Therefore, it is indisputable that opioids are not a satisfactory solution for managing chronic pain over an extended period, primarily because the mental and emotional aspects cannot be medicated.

Quotes To Spark
Thought And Discussion

"The irony of opioids is that they can make pain worse, even as they mask it."

- Jane Ballantyne, professor of anesthesiology and pain medicine at the University of Washington School of Medicine

"Opioids are a cruel joke played on us by our bodies."

- Sam Quinones, author of "Dreamland: The True Tale of America's Opiate Epidemic"

"The irony of opioids is that they can make you feel better in the short term, but they often end up making everything worse in the long term."

- Johann Hari, author of "Chasing the Scream: The First and Last Days of the War on Drugs."

"Although tolerance, dependence, and addiction are related concepts, they aren't the same. Tolerance and dependence are expected consequences of chronic opioid use, whereas addiction is a potentially unpredictable and destructive outcome."

-Nora Volkow, neuroscientist and psychiatrist,
Director of the National Institute on Drug Abuse (NIDA)

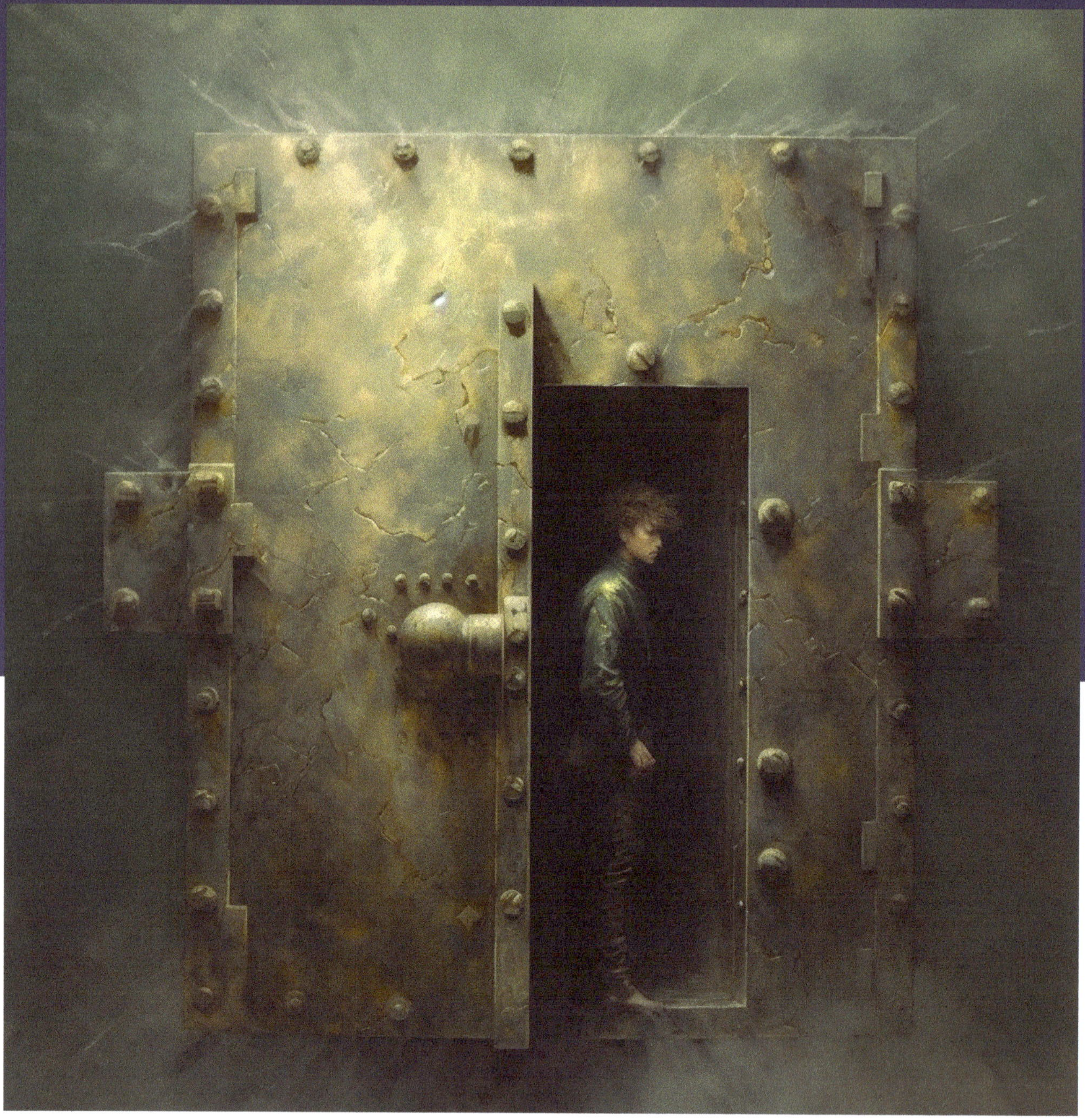

Chapter Ten

Interrelated and Distinct

Tolerance, Dependence, Addiction

What's the difference?

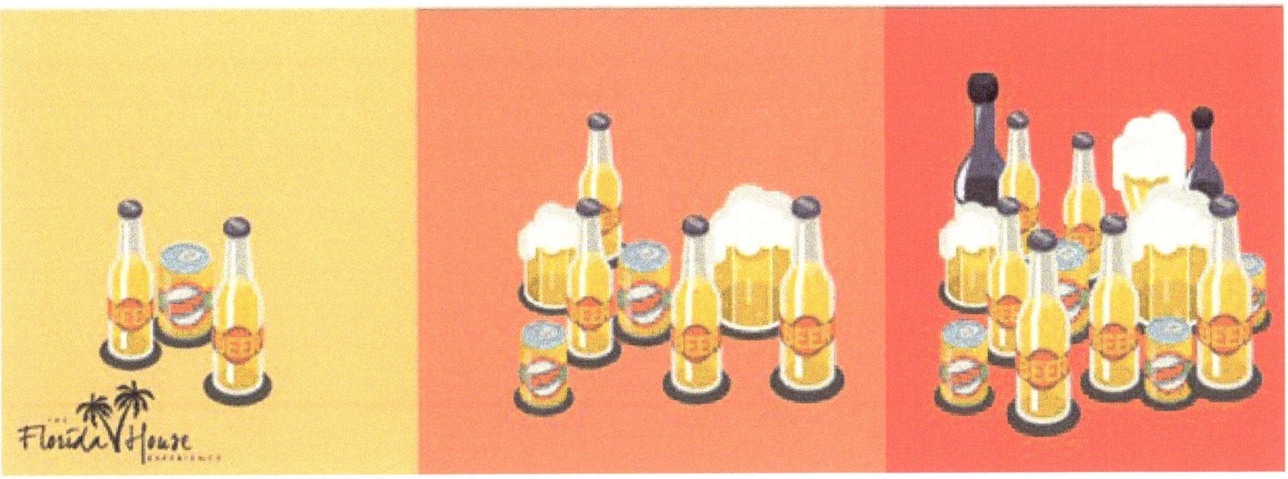

Nora Volkow, the Director of the National Institute on Drug Abuse (NIDA), highlights that although tolerance and dependence are anticipated results of persistent opioid use, addiction can be an unforeseeable and harmful consequence. Despite often being used interchangeably in conversations about opioid use, the terms "tolerance," "dependence," and "addiction" are distinct concepts that need to be distinguished. Consequently, individuals who suffer from chronic pain may feel stigmatized, or trapped, by being labeled as addicts, when most likely, this may not be the case.

Tolerance (Physical adaptation)

Tolerance is a physiological phenomenon characterized by the body's decreasing responsiveness to the effects of a drug over time. As a result, an individual requires larger doses of the drug to achieve the same effect previously achieved with a smaller dose.

This phenomenon is often seen with chronic use of medications or drugs of abuse, and it can have significant implications for the effectiveness and safety of these substances. [64]

In the brain, tolerance is thought to result from a variety of adaptive changes that occur in response to chronic drug exposure. One key factor is the down-regulation of neurotransmitter receptors, particularly those associated with the brain's reward system.

When a drug is taken repeatedly, the brain responds by reducing the number of receptors available to bind to the drug, which reduces the drug's effect on the brain's reward circuitry. This means that a larger amount of the drug is required to produce the same level of reward or pleasure that was previously achieved with a smaller amount.[65]

In addition to changes in neurotransmitter receptors, other adaptations can also contribute to tolerance. For example, the liver increases its enzymes to break down the drug, making it less effective. The kidneys may also increase their excretion of the drug, reducing the amount that remains in the bloodstream and reaches the brain[66]

Tolerance is a complex process involving changes in multiple systems throughout the body. While it can be an expected consequence of some medications, it can also be a sign of problematic drug use contributing to the development of dependence and possible addiction.

Understanding the mechanisms that underlie substance tolerance is an important area of research, as it may ultimately lead to more effective treatments for drug abuse and addiction.

Dependence (Physical Need)

Substance dependence refers to the physical reliance on a drug that is characterized by the development of tolerance, withdrawal symptoms upon cessation of drug use, and a persistent desire to continue using the substance despite adverse consequences.[6] It is also commonly known as "physical dependence" because it involves changes in the body's chemistry and functioning that lead to a physical reliance on the drug to function normally.[67][68]

It is VITAL to differentiate between substance dependence and addiction! They are interrelated and distinct.

Addiction is a more comprehensive term that includes both physical and psychological dependence. Psychological dependence involves the emotional and behavioral aspects of addiction, such as the compulsion to use drugs to cope with stress or to experience pleasure.

Addiction involves both physical and psychological components, and it is characterized by compulsive drug use despite negative consequences, as well as a loss of control over drug use.[69]

In summary, while substance dependence refers to physical reliance on a drug, addiction includes both physical and psychological dependence, characterized by compulsive drug use and a loss of control.

Addiction (Mental/Lifestyle)

Misconceptions surrounding substance dependence and addiction have fueled the stigma around patients with chronic pain. While substance dependence and addiction are related, they are not the same.[70]

As stated, dependence refers to a physical state in which the body has adapted to a drug, requiring a certain amount to avoid withdrawal symptoms. Addiction is a complex and chronic condition characterized by compulsive drug use despite negative consequences.[71]

While tolerance and dependence are not necessarily problematic in and of themselves, they can contribute to the development of addiction. For example, as individuals develop tolerance to opioids, they may take higher doses to achieve the same effect, which can increase the risk of overdose. Similarly, dependence can lead to withdrawal symptoms that motivate continued drug use, even in the face of negative consequences.[72]

It is essential to differentiate between substance dependence and addiction to provide appropriate treatment and prevent the stigmatization of patients with chronic pain. Making that distinction can help avoid worsening the situation for those living with chronic pain.

While all addicted individuals are dependent on substances, most individuals who take medications are not addicted!

In summary, tolerance, dependence, and addiction are distinct but interrelated concepts that should be clearly distinguished in discussions about and with patients with chronic pain and opioid use therapy. Although these terms are often used interchangeably, it is important to understand their unique features and implications to ensure effective prevention, destroy the stigma, and create unique treatment strategies for opioid-related problems.

Quotes To Spark
Thought And Discussion

"Tolerance is a physical phenomenon where the body adapts to the presence of a substance over time, requiring greater amounts to achieve the same effects. Dependence is a psychological phenomenon where the body becomes used to the presence of a substance and experiences withdrawal symptoms when the substance is removed. Addiction is a complex disease characterized by compulsive drug seeking and use despite harmful consequences."

-National Institute on Drug Abuse

"Tolerance is a natural process that occurs with regular use of many drugs. Dependence is a state where the body relies on a drug to prevent withdrawal symptoms. Addiction is a disorder characterized by compulsive drug seeking and use despite negative consequences."

- Nora Volkow

“Tolerance is the capacity of the body to accommodate the substance. Dependence is the adaptation of the organism to the substance. Addiction is the taking of a substance to relieve stress or emotional pain.”

- Gabor Maté

“Tolerance is a predictable response to repeated drug use that requires increased dosages to achieve the same effect. Dependence is the body’s physical adaptation to the drug, requiring continued use to prevent withdrawal symptoms. Addiction is a chronic and relapsing brain disease characterized by compulsive drug-seeking behavior despite the harmful consequences.”

- American Society of Addiction Medicine

”Tolerance is the body’s adaptation to a substance, requiring more to achieve the same effect. Dependence is the body’s reliance on a substance, leading to withdrawal symptoms when the substance is discontinued. Addiction is the inability to stop using a substance despite negative consequences.”

- Dr. Judson Brewer

"The problem with opioids is that they create a pain cycle, where the more you take, the more pain you have, and the more you need to take to treat the pain."

-Dr. Forest Tennant, a pain management specialist and addiction expert

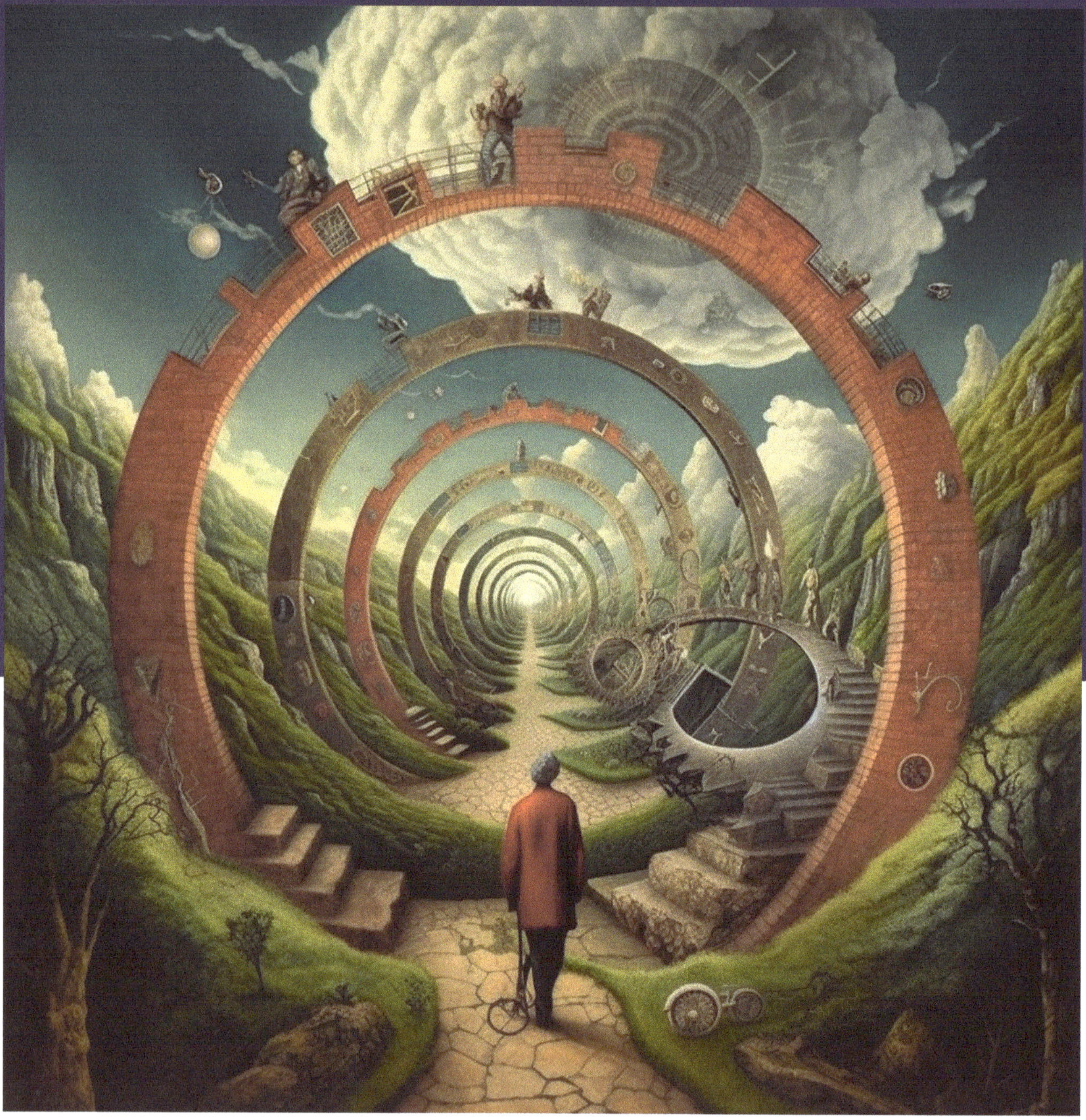

Chapter Eleven

Paradoxical Dependence

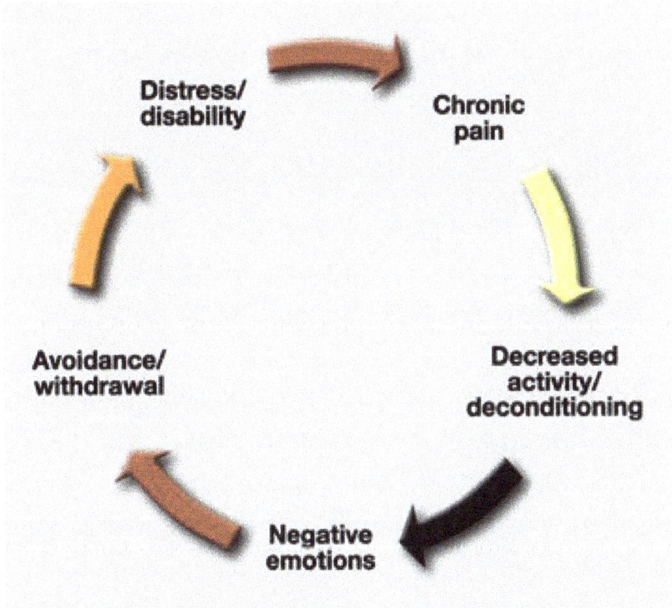

Chronic pain is a debilitating and paradoxical condition that can significantly affect a person's quality of life. For many patients with chronic pain, the pain is not just physical, but also psychological, as it can lead to a vicious cycle of negative emotions and lifestyle disability.

- *The first step* in this cycle is sensing pain. Patients with chronic pain often experience pain that is persistent and does not respond to traditional pain management strategies.
- *The second step* is that pain leads to decreased activity as patients cannot perform daily activities, work, or engage in recreational activities. The decreased activity, in turn, can lead to feelings of frustration, anxiety, and depression.[73]
- *The third step* is that negative emotions associated with chronic pain can lead to…
- *The fourth step* is avoidance behaviors. Patients may avoid certain activities or situations that they perceive as causing or exacerbating their pain. For example, a patient with chronic back pain may avoid bending or lifting heavy objects, leading to further de-conditioning and decreased physical activity.[74] Avoidance behaviors can then lead to the…
- *Fifth and final step* of lifestyle distress/disability. Chronic pain patients may become increasingly isolated and withdrawn, which can impact their social relationships, employment opportunities, and overall quality of life. Over time, this can lead to a sense of helplessness and hopelessness, perpetuating the cycle of chronic pain and negative emotions.[75]

When we realize we're in a rut like this; what do we do about it? The trick to arresting the cycle is all in the timing, as Amanda Wakefield explains:

"The distress/disability phase of the pain cycle is the most amenable (easiest) to change in therapy. It's harder to intervene in the sensing pain phase.This is because pain is directly influenced by mood, activity level, etc., and can vary widely.

Activities or attitudes can directly intervene in the cycle in other areas, and they will indirectly affect pain. A therapist uses models like these to identify the impact of actions (or lack of action) in a certain area of functioning. This cycle is especially relevant to people who are not doing enough activity.

All areas can be used for intervention and are used frequently. I find that chronic pain is the hardest to intervene in. However, teaching appropriate pacing can be a powerful direct intervention even in this phase. Sometimes it works best to identify the areas a patient already believes have the most potential for change and start there."

Chronic pain is a challenging condition that can have profound physical and emotional impacts on patients. The "wind-up effect", a phenomenon where pain signals become amplified and the brain becomes more sensitive to pain over time, leads to a cycle of increased pain perception, reduced activity, negative emotions, avoidance, and lifestyle disability.

This cycle can be difficult to break, highlighting the need for a multidisciplinary approach to chronic pain management. The SHRP Approach is one example, emphasizing the integration of medical, behavioral, and physical therapies to improve patient outcomes and enhance their overall quality of life.

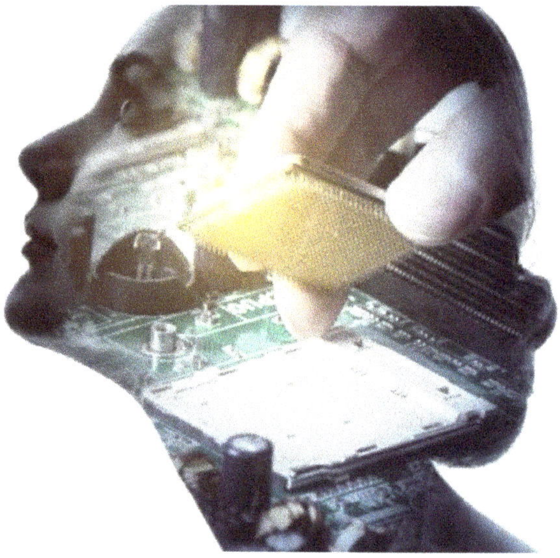

Quotes To Spark
Thought And Discussion

*"The wind-up effect is like a cruel joke.
The more you feel pain,
the more pain you feel."*

- Dr. Beth Darnall, a pain psychologist and researcher at Stanford University.

"Chronic pain is a vicious cycle, where the brain's natural response to pain amplifies the pain signal, leading to more pain and suffering."

- Dr. Daniel Clauw, Director of the Chronic Pain, and Fatigue Research Center at the University of Michigan.

*"The irony of chronic pain is that the more you try to fight it, the worse it can get.
It's like quicksand, the more you struggle, the deeper you sink."*

- Karen Duffy, author and chronic pain advocate.

"To interrupt chronic pain and wind down the wind-up effect, a person must attend to his or her physical, mental, emotional, and spiritual needs, as this creates a healthy tension that fosters creativity."

-Glenn Banks

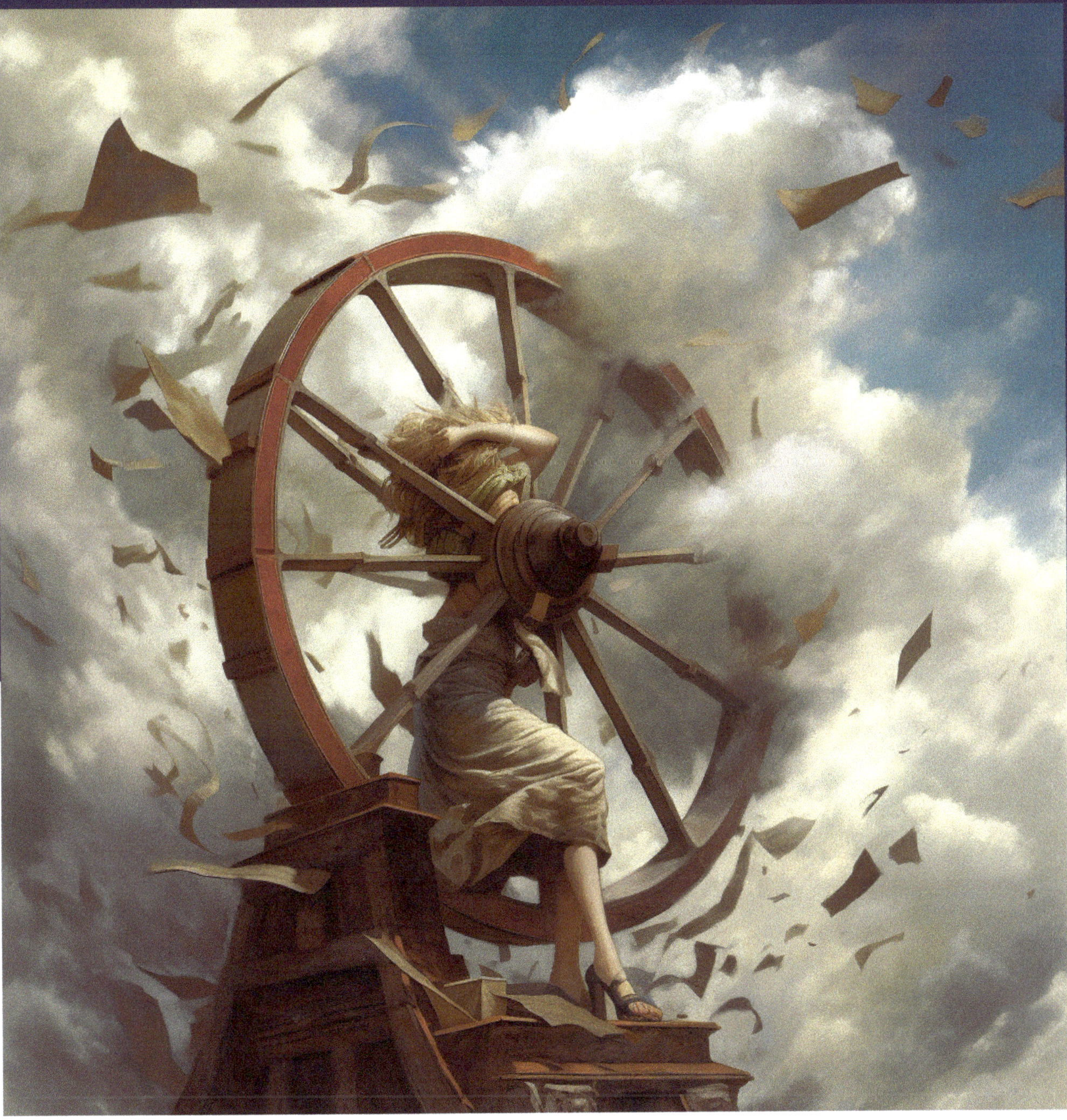

Chapter Twelve

Breaking the Pain Cycle

The SHRP plan recognizes the importance of an interdisciplinary approach to managing chronic pain. Its main goal is to improve patients' quality of life and outcomes by prioritizing the integration of medical, behavioral, and physical therapies.

However, adding to these therapeutic interventions, it's essential to understand that meeting our fundamental human needs is the foundation for achieving overall well-being and reducing the wind-up effect.

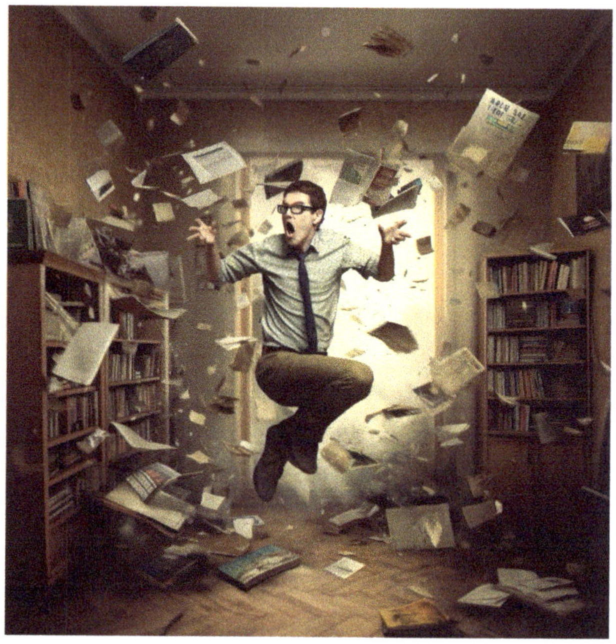

As Amanda explained above, "...to identify the areas a patient already believes have the most potential for change and start there." We achieve this by building creative tension. Creative tension is the mental and emotional discomfort or stress that arises when we have a vision or goal not aligned with our current reality.

We build creative tension by setting challenging and achievable goals and working toward them, helping us to stay motivated and focused.

This can involve developing a clear vision of what we want to achieve, creating a plan to get there, regularly reflecting on our progress, and adjusting as needed. By building creative tension, we move toward a more fulfilling and satisfying life, reducing chronic pain.

In his book, "***The Path of Least Resistance***," Robert Fritz explains that creative tension can be built by having a clear vision of a desired outcome or goal and comparing that vision to the current reality or situation [76]

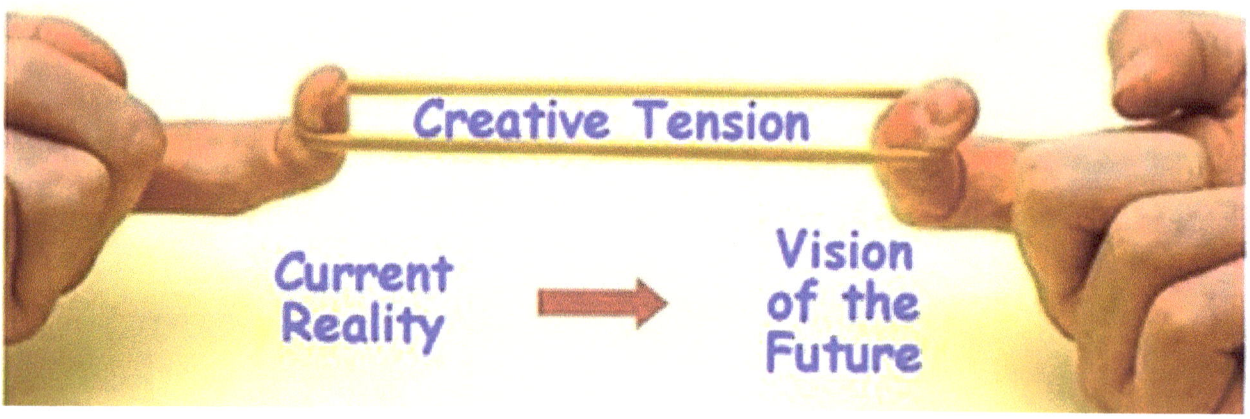

The gap between the vision and current reality creates a tension that drives the individual to act and make changes to achieve the desired outcome. By continuously adjusting and refining the vision, and acting toward accomplishing it, creative tension is maintained, and progress is made towards the goal.

It is common for chronic pain patients to be consumed by their pain and its effects, making it challenging for them to consider a vision for managing their pain. Many may not have been exposed to the idea of creative tension or have had access to resources and support to help them develop a vision. Additionally, chronic pain can be an overwhelming issue, making it difficult for individuals to envision a path forward.

Robert Fritz suggests that individuals with a good current reality but lack vision may become stagnant and unmotivated. Conversely, those with a vision but no clear understanding of their current reality may feel overwhelmed and discouraged, leading to a lack of motivation to act towards their desired outcome.

Therefore, it is necessary to understand one's current reality to effectively plan and act toward achieving a vision. To increase an understanding of one's current reality, Fritz advises observing and analyzing the situation by paying attention to thoughts, emotions, and behaviors, and seeking feedback from others.

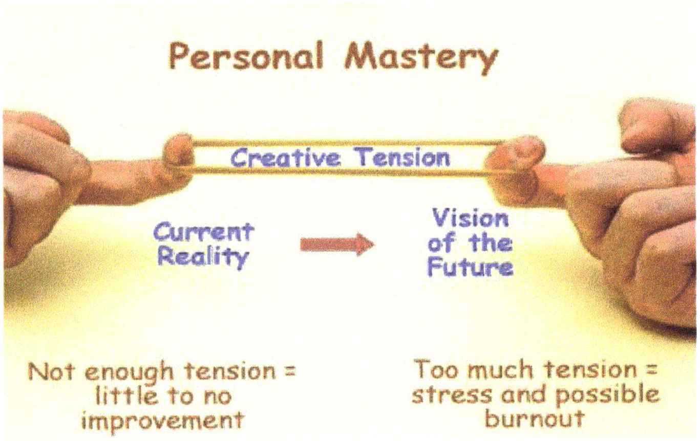

Once people grasp their current reality, they can develop a vision for their desired outcome and build creative tension to achieve it.

Fritz suggests exploring and experimenting with different possibilities for those without a vision. Individuals can engage in activities that spark curiosity and passion, seek new experiences and perspectives to expand their understanding of what is possible, and find what resonates with them.

Please complete the Creative Tension Exercise on the next page:

Creative Tension Exercise

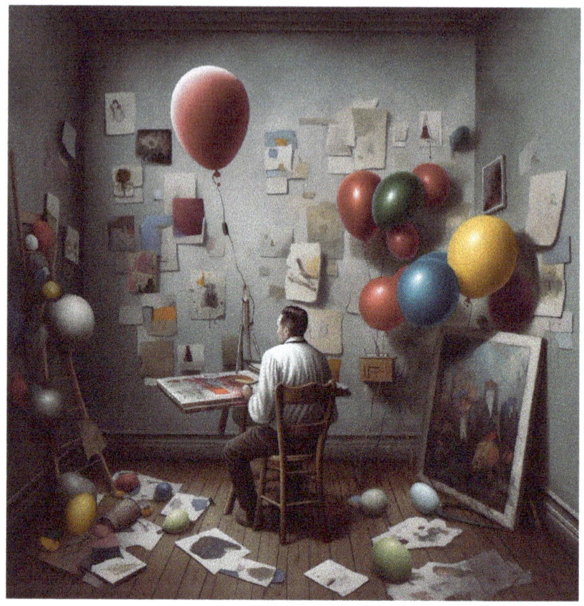

Consider documenting or discussing with a trusted individual how well you are currently managing your chronic pain situation ***(Current reality):***

Consider documenting or having a conversation with a trusted individual regarding your clearly defined outcome for effectively managing your chronic pain situation in the future ***(Vision):***

The Creative Tension Exercise helps patients with chronic pain understand their current situation while envisioning a future that inspires and motivates them to pursue their goals.

In the following chapter, the SHRP Guide is introduced as a useful tool for developing "creative tension" by identifying and fulfilling important human needs in five essential areas: spirituality, belonging, variety, importance, and basic needs.

By utilizing this guide, individuals with chronic pain have clarity on their current reality and develop a vision that drives them toward their desired outcomes.

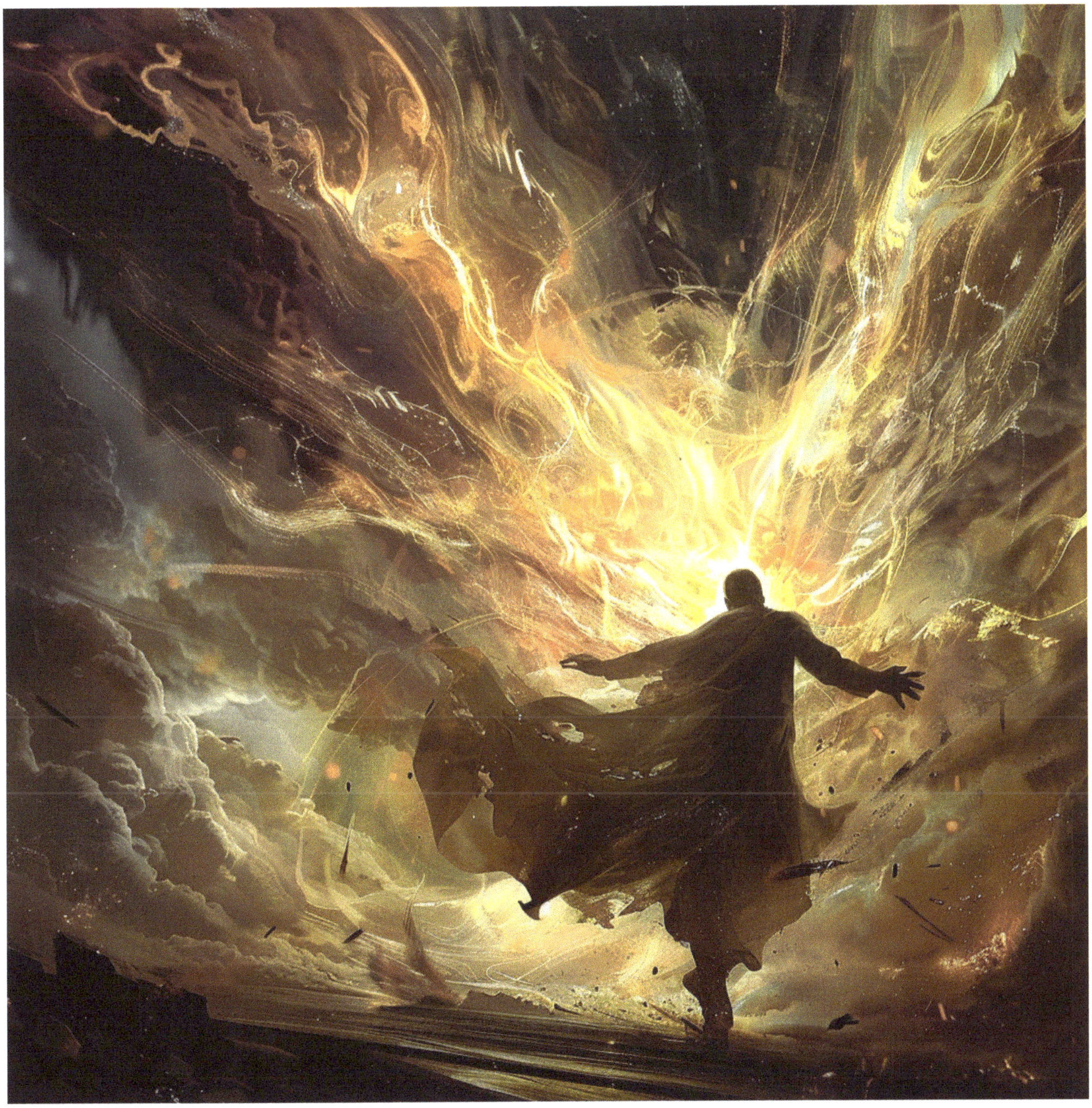

"The deeper the sense of personal responsibility and purpose or meaning in life, the greater the overall sense of well-being and health."

-Carl Jung

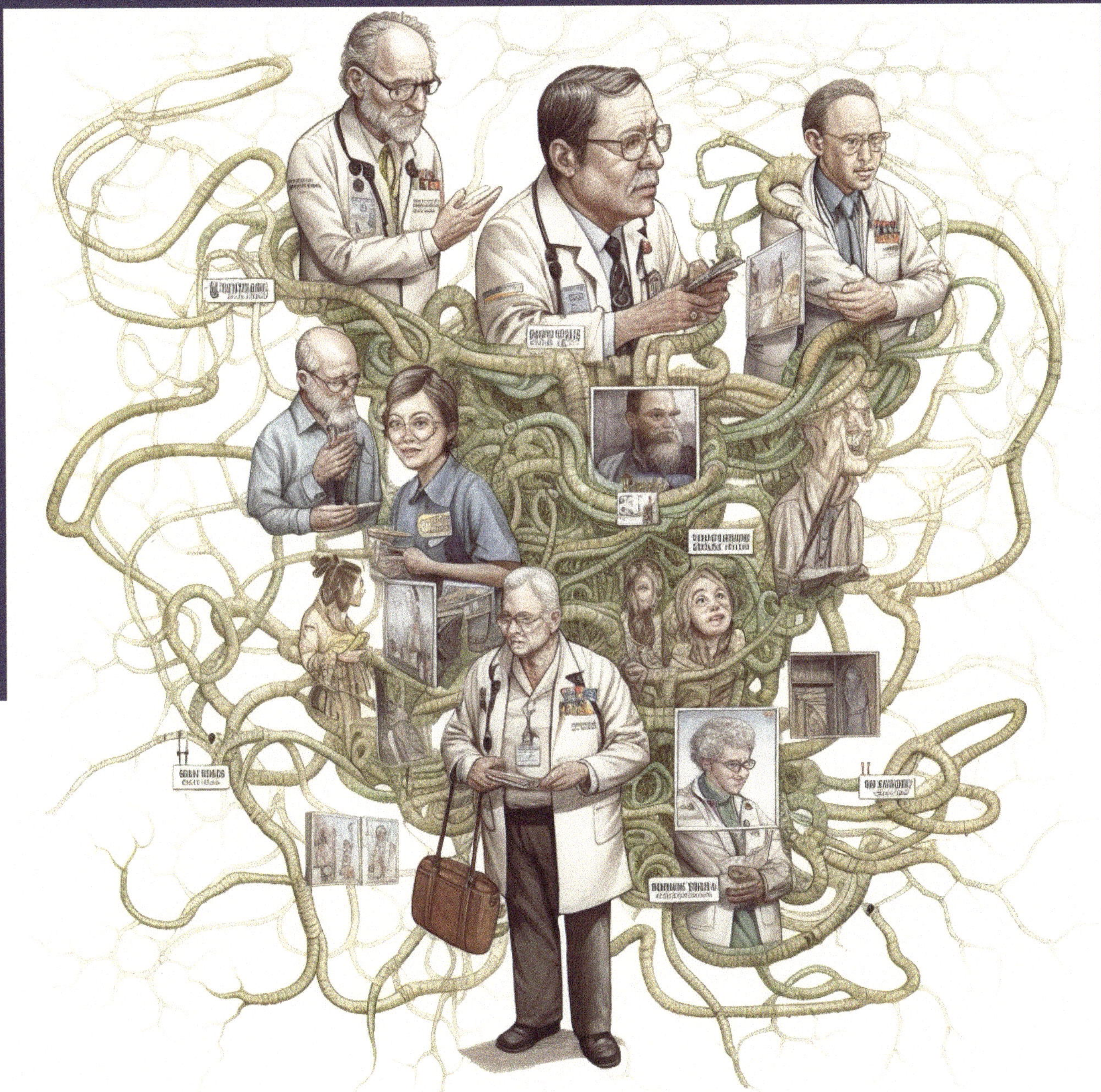

Chapter Thirteen

The Strategic Harm Reduction Plan (SHRP)

According to research in positive psychology, assuming a sense of purpose and being accountable for one's actions can substantially enhance mental and physical well-being. The fundamental principle of the SHRP approach accentuates the significance of continually endeavoring to "keep our brain sensing safety" by satisfying our diverse needs, such as spiritual, social, variety, significance, and fundamental requirements. This is deemed a vital personal obligation for managing chronic pain. The diagram below visually shows this idea.

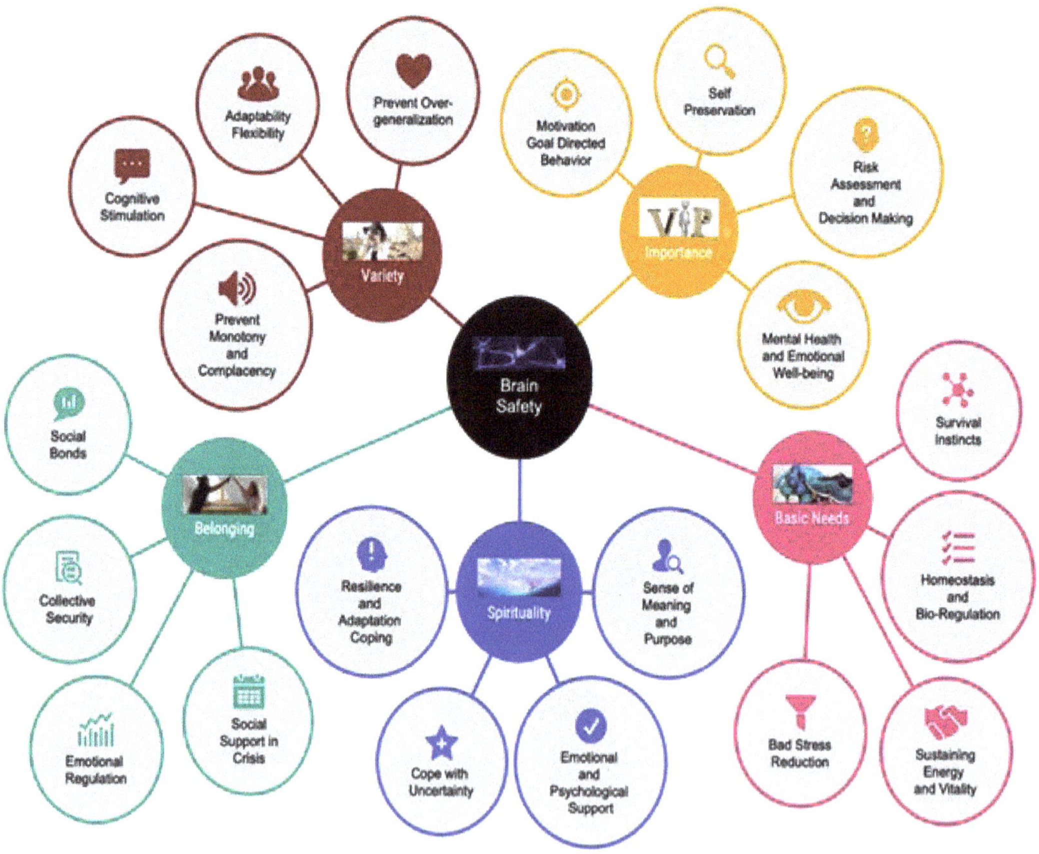

Spirituality Need

Spirituality can serve as a trustworthy source of information to help us answer life's questions. When our brain can answer the fundamental questions of who, what, where, when, why, and how to minimize perceived threats, it can help to calm us and "wind us down".

The wind-up effect refers to accumulating stress and anxiety over time, leading to feeling overwhelmed, burnt out, or emotionally exhausted. Engaging in daily spiritual practices, such as pondering on personal relevant questions of life, has been proven to help lower the wind-up effect by providing a sense of purpose, meaning, and connection to something greater than oneself (the brain feels safer).

Several words are like spirituality, including:

Faith, religion, belief, mysticism, transcendence, devotion, philosophy, metaphysics, esotericism, and theology.

Each word relates to a belief system or way of understanding the world beyond the material or physical realm. They all involve some form of connection to a higher power or purpose and a belief in something greater than oneself.

While there are differences in meaning and connotation, they are all related to spirituality.

Here are some examples of basic life questions:

- What is the purpose of my life?
- What do I value most in life?
- What are my long-term goals?
- What are my short-term goals?
- What brings me happiness and fulfillment?
- What are my strengths and weaknesses?
- How can I improve myself?

- What is my definition of success?
- What legacy do I want to leave behind?
- What is my relationship with others?
- What is my relationship with nature?
- What is my relationship with the divine or spiritual?
- What is my philosophy of life?
- What do I believe happens after death?

These are just a few examples of basic life questions. There are many other questions that one could ask oneself to gain insight and clarity about life and purpose.

When we engage in daily spiritual practices, we tap into our inner wisdom and intuition, which can help us gain clarity and perspective on our life circumstances. By reflecting on our life's questions, we gain insight into our values, beliefs, and goals, which can help us prioritize our time and energy in a way that aligns with our authentic selves.

Daily spiritual practices also often involve mindfulness and meditation, which can help us cultivate a sense of calm and inner peace. By focusing on the present moment and letting go of worries about the future or regrets about the past, our brain senses safety, and the brain can reduce the amount of stress, anxiety, and pain we experience. Increasing spirituality is a highly personal and subjective process.

Here are some suggested examples of practices that people have found helpful in enhancing their spiritual connection:

- Meditation and mindfulness practices
- Prayer or spiritual ritual
- Spending time in nature or practicing eco-spirituality.
- Reading and reflecting on sacred texts or spiritual literature
- Practicing gratitude and compassion towards oneself and others
- Engaging in community service or volunteer work

- Cultivating meaningful relationships and connections with others
- Attending religious or spiritual services or gatherings
- Practicing yoga or other forms of movement meditation
- Creating art or engaging in other creative activities as a form of expression and connection with the divine.

It's important to note that what works for one person may not work for another. Exploring different practices and finding what resonates with our unique spiritual journey is essential.

Daily spirituality practices help our brain answer our current personal life questions through a spiritual connection. Strengthening this connection helps us manage the wind-up effect by providing a sense of purpose, clarity, meaning, and inner peace. By making space for daily spiritual practices, we can cultivate resilience, reduce stress, and reduce our wind-up effect.

Ask yourself these questions:

What does spirituality mean to me? What spiritual practices do I engage in regularly, if any? How can I incorporate more spirituality into my life to help me answer life's questions better and improve my overall well-being, thus taking control of my wind-up effect?

Answer here:

Answer here:

Honestly think about this next question:

How well am I meeting my spiritual needs on a scale from 1 to 10? (10 being the best)

If your spiritual need score is a "10":

Congratulations! Your spirit is soaring higher than a bald eagle on the fourth of July! Your connection to the divine is so strong, it's like you have a direct line to the heavens. You're probably meditating like a boss, manifesting your dreams into reality, and radiating so much positive energy, people mistake you for a walking sunbeam. Your aura is sparkling like a diamond in the sunlight, and your chakras are spinning like a disco ball on New Year's Eve. You're a true spiritual ninja, with the power to transform yourself and the world around you. So go ahead and do your happydance, because you've earned it! Just remember to stay grounded, stay humble, and keep spreading that light to those who need it most. Namaste!

If your spirituality need score is a "1":

It means your spiritual life needs serious CPR (Cosmic Power Resuscitation)! You might feel like a lost soul, wandering in the wilderness of your thoughts, wondering if there's any meaning to your existence beyond Netflix and chill. You're probably not on speaking terms with your inner guru, and your chakras are so blocked, that they could double as a parking lot. But fear not, for even the most enlightened beings had to start somewhere, and with a little effort, you too can rekindle the flame of your inner spirit and embark on a journey of self-discovery and transcendence. So put on your soul-searching boots, grab your prayer beads, and get this spiritual party started!

Rate your answer with a score below.

Spirituality Score (1-10):

___

Belonging Need

Meeting your human belonging needs helps to lower the wind-up effect by providing a sense of connection and support from others. Humans are social beings and feeling a sense of belonging and connection with others, is a fundamental need for our well-being. When this need is met, it can help to reduce stress and anxiety and promote feelings of security and safety.

Meeting this need also increases resilience and ability to cope with challenges, by providing a network of social support and resources we can draw upon during difficult times. This helps to bring down the wind-up effect, reduce the negative impact of stress on our body and mind, and promote overall health and well-being.

Loneliness ranks among the top three reasons the wind-up effect holds such power over us. It is a negative experience for humans, bringing isolation, disconnection, and sadness. Loneliness leads us to believe that we cannot connect with others or have meaningful relationships, creating a sense of hopelessness, helplessness, and despair, all contributing to the wind-up effect.

In addition to its emotional effects, loneliness can also have adverse physical effects on the body, including elevated stress hormone levels, inflammation, and a weakened immune system. These physiological changes can further increase vulnerability to negative emotions and stress, reinforcing the wind-up effect.

It's important to note that loneliness and being alone are not the same things. It is possible to be alone and feel content and fulfilled, while loneliness is a subjective feeling of social isolation and disconnection.

By building meaningful relationships and connecting with others, we can experience a sense of belonging and purpose that can help to lower the wind-up effect. Several words are like belonging, including:

Inclusion, community, membership, fellowship, association, unity, solidarity, connection, relationship, and affiliation.

These words relate to being part of a group or community and feeling a sense of connectedness and belongingness. They all involve feeling welcomed and accepted by others and a shared identity or purpose.

While there are some differences in meaning and connotation between these words, they are all related to the concept of belonging in some way.

Here are a few examples of how to get our human belonging needs met:

- Joining a club or group that shares your interests or hobbies.
- Attending social events and gatherings with family and friends
- Participating in team sports or other group activities
- Volunteering for a cause you care about
- Joining a religious or spiritual community
- Connecting with others through online communities or social media groups
- Joining a support group for people with shared experiences or challenges
- Participating in group therapy or counseling sessions
- Engaging in conversations with colleagues or classmates
- Building and maintaining close relationships with family, friends, or romantic partners.

Finding individuals, activities, and/or communities that align with your values and interests, allowing you to connect with others, is essential. By doing so, you can satisfy your human belonging need and experience the many benefits of social connection and support.

Ask yourself these questions:

Who are the people in my life who provide me with a sense of belonging? How can I deepen my connection with these individuals and/or expand my social support network? What community resources are available to me that can provide me a sense of belonging (e.g., support groups, clubs, volunteering)?

Answer here:

Honestly think about this next question:

How well am I meeting my belonging needs on a scale from 1 to 10? (10 being the best)?

If your belonging need score is a "10":

Congratulations! You're as socially connected as a Kardashian at a red-carpet event. You have more friends than you can count on both hands and feet, and your phone constantly buzzes with messages and notifications from your social circle. Your Instagram feed looks like a highlight reel of your epic adventures and social events, and your LinkedIn network is a who's who of movers and shakers in your industry. You strike conversations with anyone, anywhere, and your charisma is more powerful than a Jedi mind trick. So go ahead, bask in the glow of your social prowess, and keep spreading those good vibes wherever you go!

If your belonging need score is a "1":

It means you're about as connected to others as a hermit crab living in an abandoned seashell. You might feel stuck in a social desert, with no oasis in sight. Your Facebook friend list looks more like a ghost town, and the last time you had a meaningful conversation with someone was during the solar eclipse. Your idea of social interaction is probably limited to yelling at the TV during a game show, and your social skills are about as polished as a rock in a river. With a little effort and creative thinking, you too could find your tribe and start building meaningful connections with others. So put on your social butterfly wings, grab a few conversation starters, and start the party!

Rate your answer with a score below.

Belonging Score (1-10):

____

Variety Need

Meeting your human variety needs lowers the wind-up effect by providing opportunities for novelty and variety. When you engage in new experiences, try new things, and expose yourself to different perspectives, you activate your brain's reward center and release feel-good chemicals like dopamine.

This can help counteract the stress response and reduce the negative impact of the wind-up effect. Moreover, having diverse social connections and exposure to different cultures, opinions, and lifestyles broadens your perspective and helps you develop more adaptable and flexible ways of thinking.

This can help you better cope with challenging situations and reduce the likelihood of getting stuck in negative patterns of thought and behavior.

Overall, meeting your human variety needs can be an effective way to reduce the wind-up effect and enhance your overall well-being. Here are some other words that can connote variety, including:

Passion, excitement, thrill, adventure, novelty, diversity, stimulation, passion, interest, curiosity, and enthusiasm.

These words connote a sense of liveliness, passion, and interest that can help counteract boredom and monotony. They all relate to experiencing new things, exploring different options, and feeling energized by the world.

While some of these words may have slightly different meanings or connotations, they share a common thread conveying a sense of variety and engagement.

Boredom is one of the top three reasons why the wind-up effect can have such a strong hold on us. This is because boredom harms our well-being, leading to feelings of disengagement, apathy, and dissatisfaction with life.

When bored, we may feel like we are not experiencing anything new or meaningful, which can contribute to a sense of stagnation or even despair.

Additionally, boredom can make us more vulnerable to negative emotions such as stress, anxiety, and depression, as we may feel like we are not fulfilling our potential or that our lives lack purpose.

Boredom can fuel the wind-up effect by elevating our stress and anxiety levels. When we experience boredom, our minds may gravitate towards pessimistic thoughts and concerns, and feel "unsafe", resulting in mental and emotional strain.

Gradually, this strain can escalate, causing our brains to perceive a sense of insecurity, and inducing a heightened state of arousal that impairs our ability to cope with stress and anxiety.

In essence, boredom triggers the wind-up effect, amplifying our susceptibility to harmful "unsafe" thoughts and emotions, thus initiating a perpetual cycle of tension and stress over time.

Ask yourself these questions:

What are some activities that I enjoy doing in my free time? Do I incorporate more variety into my life to prevent boredom and increase enjoyment? Are there new activities or hobbies I have been interested in trying but have not yet pursued? If so, what steps can I take to try them out?

Answer here:

Honestly think about this next question:

How well am I meeting my variety needs on a scale from 1 to 10? (10 being the best)?

If your variety need score is a "10":

It would be like having a personal assistant whose only job is to randomly generate new and exciting experiences for you every day. One day, you might find yourself skydiving over the Grand Canyon, while the next day you might be learning to tango in Argentina or taking part in a cooking class in Thailand. You would constantly be exposed to new cultures, ideas, and activities, and your life would be a non-stop adventure. You might even start to feel a bit like a character from a James Bond movie, always on the move and ready for the next big thing.

If your variety need score is a "1":

It would be like living in a world where everything is beige. Your wardrobe would consist of only one color, your meals would consist of only one type of food, and your entertainment would consist of only one TV channel. Every day would be the same, and there would be no room for spontaneity or excitement. You might start to feel like a character in the movie Groundhog Day, living the same day repeatedly, with nothing new or interesting to break up the monotony. The only variety you might experience would be the occasional dust bunny rolling across your beige carpet.

Rate your answer with a score below.

Variety Score (1-10):

____

Importance Need

Meeting our human importance needs lowers the wind-up effect in several ways. We feel valued and appreciated by others, it boosts our self-esteem and increases our sense of self-worth. This leads to greater control over our lives and emotions, decreasing stress and anxiety.

Additionally, when we feel important, we are more likely to engage in meaningful activities and provide a sense of purpose and fulfillment that counteracts the negative effects of stress and tension.

Meeting our human importance needs increases our social support network and provides a buffer against stress and anxiety. When we have people who value and support us, we feel more comfortable seeking help and support when we need it. This helps us to manage stress more effectively and prevent the wind-up effect from taking hold.

Feeling important is a subjective experience and varies from person to person. However, here are some general things that people do to boost their sense of importance:

- ***Set goals:*** Setting achievable goals and working towards them can give a sense of purpose and accomplishment, which makes a person feel important.
- ***Volunteer:*** Helping others and contributing to society can give a sense of purpose and significance.
- ***Learn something new:*** Acquiring new knowledge or skills can make a person feel more confident and capable, contributing to a sense of importance.
- ***Exercise:*** Regular exercise has been shown to boost self-esteem and confidence, which can increase feelings of importance.
- ***Practice self-care:*** Taking care of oneself, whether through mindfulness meditation, getting enough sleep, or treating oneself to something nice, promotes a sense of self-worth and importance.
- ***Surround oneself with positive people:*** Being around supportive and positive people helps a person feel valued and important.
- ***Celebrate accomplishments:*** Recognizing and celebrating personal achievements, no matter how small, contributes to a sense of importance and accomplishment.

Overall, meeting our human importance needs provides a sense of validation, purpose, and social support that can help lower the wind-up effect and promote greater emotional well-being. Here are some other words that convey a similar meaning to importance:

Significance, relevance, meaningfulness, prestige,prominence, distinction, worth, influence, and impact.

These words connote a sense of importance, relevance, or significance. They are often used to describe something that has a meaningful impact or carries weight and value in a particular context.

Some of these words, such as "significance" and "meaningfulness," imply a deeper, more philosophical, or emotional sense of importance, while others, such as "value" and "prominence," may have more concrete or practical implications.

Ask yourself these questions:

Do I have a purpose or a sense of meaning in my life? Do I feel like I have the power to make choices and decisions that affect my life and those around me? Am I making a positive impact in the world, no matter how small? Do I feel like I am contributing to something greater than myself?

Answer here:

Honestly think about this next question:

How well am I meeting my importance needs on a scale from 1 to 10? (10 being the best)?

If your importance need score is a "10":

It would seem like you were the ruler of the universe, with all beings at your beck and call, and the stars themselves spelling out your name in the night sky. You would be so important that your mere presence causes a rush of excitement in anyone who sees you, and your every word would be considered gospel truth. In short, you would be the ultimate boss of everything and everyone, and no one would dare to cross you!

If your importance need score is a "1":

You would be like the world's smallest fish in the world's largest ocean. In other words, your significance would be almost non-existent. It would be like a grain of sand on a beach or a single drop of water in a vast ocean. You would feel so insignificant that even ants would look down on you.Or it would be like a pebble in a shoe, you might be annoying but ultimately irrelevant.

Rate your answer with a score below.

Importance Score (1-10):

____

Basic Needs

Meeting our basic needs means fulfilling the essential requirements for survival and well-being, not just food, water, shelter, and clothing, but sex, sleep, exercise, and nutritional health.

Maslow's Hierarchy of Needs describes how fulfilling our physiological and safety needs are fundamental to human survival, followed by our psychological and social needs, and finally our self-actualization needs.

When our basic needs are met, the brain is less likely to feel "unsafe" because our bodies and minds are not preoccupied with survival concerns. This helps to manage the wind-up effect because we are not in a constant state of heightened arousal, which contributes to the wind-up effect for chronic pain patients.

Research suggests that when individuals have their basic needs met, they are more likely to experience a sense of safety and security, decreasing the wind-up effect.

For example, a study published in the Journal of Social and Clinical Psychology found that individuals who reported experiencing food insecurity had higher levels of anxiety and depression compared to those who did not experience food insecurity.[77]

Additionally, a report by the National Law Center on Homelessness and Poverty found that individuals experiencing homelessness had higher levels of stress, anxiety, and depression compared to those with stable housing.[78]

Moreover, trauma-informed care research has shown that individuals are less likely to feel anxious or angry when their bodies are fully relaxed.[79] This suggests that when individuals have their basic needs met and feel safe, their bodies can relax, decreasing stress and anxiety, and the winding down of their nervous system.

Therefore, fulfilling basic needs such as access to nutritious food, safe shelter, sleep, sex, exercise, etc., effectively manages the wind-up effect.

As stated, the wind-up effect refers to the phenomenon where repeated exposure to painful stimuli can cause an individual to become more sensitive to pain over time, which can stabilize or increase pain even though healing has occurred. Research has shown that the number one key factor contributing to increasing wind-up effect (more pain) is immobility, which refers to being physically inactive or sedentary.

Studies have found that immobility can increase the wind-up effect by causing changes in the central nervous system, including the brain and spinal cord. One study published in the Journal of Pain found that immobilization increased sensitivity to pain in healthy individuals, suggesting immobility can harm pain perception.[80]

Another study published in the journal Neuroscience Letters found that immobilization can alter the function of pain-processing neurons in the spinal cord, leading to increased pain sensitivity.[81]

In addition, immobility leads to physical changes in the body that can increase pain sensitivity. For example, when we are immobile, our muscles may become tight or tense, leading to discomfort and pain. Immobility can also lead to decreased blood flow and oxygen to the tissues, contributing to pain and discomfort.

On the other hand, physical activity has been shown to positively affect our pain perception and help reduce the wind-up effect.[82] Exercise has been found to release endorphins, natural painkillers that alleviate pain and discomfort. It helps improve blood flow and the oxygenation of tissues, promoting healing and reducing pain.

Immobility is the number one factor in increasing the wind-up effect, and can increase pain sensitivity.

Engaging in physical activity and avoiding prolonged immobility can help to reduce the wind-up effect and improve pain perception.

It is important to note that while fulfilling our basic needs is important, it does not necessarily mean that we will "feel" fulfilled or happy. Once our basic needs are met, we still need to work on fulfilling our psychological and social needs to achieve greater well-being and satisfaction in life.

Ask yourself these questions:

Do I even know what my basic needs are? Am I meeting your basic needs for food, water, sleep, sex, breathing, clothing, and shelter? Are there any barriers preventing me from meeting my basic needs? If so, what can I do to address these barriers? How am I taking care of my basic needs regularly to support my overall well-being?

Answer here:

Honestly think about this next question:

How well am I meeting my basic needs on a scale from 1 to 10? (10 being the best)?

If your basic need score is a "10":

It would look like you're living in a luxurious palace with everything you could need at your fingertips. Your bed would be made of clouds and your pillows would be stuffed with the softest feathers. Your meals would be prepared by a personal chef and served on golden plates. You would have a team of assistants to take care of all your errands and responsibilities, and you would never have to lift a finger. You'd be living like a pampered celebrity on a tropical island.

If your basic need score is a "1":

It would look like you're living in a haunted house with no electricity, no food, and no Wi-Fi. You're also being chased by a ghost, and you have no shoes, no pants, and only one sock. To make matters worse, it's raining outside, and there's a flood, so you can't escape. But hey, at least you have your trusty pet rock to keep you company!

Rate your answer with a score below.

Basic Score (1-10):

____

Write Down All Five Of Your Scores And Add Them Up:

Spirituality score: ______________________

Belonging score: ______________________

Variety score: ______________________

Importance score: ______________________

Basic Needs score: ______________________

Total SHRP Score: ______________________

This is your current SHRP Score!

Always remember that no matter where you are on your journey, there is hope for improvement if your SHRP Score is lower than anticipated. (We will discuss and interpret your SHRP Score later in Chapter 15.)

Prioritizing basic needs like food, shelter, safety, and social connections, significantly impacts your physical and emotional well-being, which can ultimately help reduce the wind-up effect.

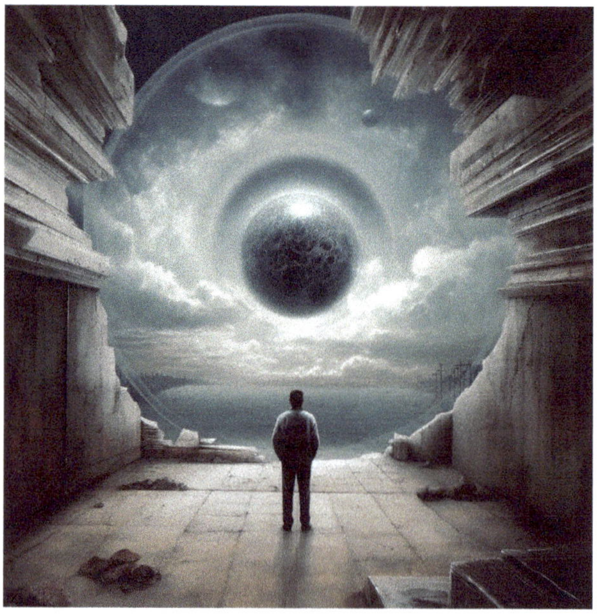

Keep going, and don't give up!

Please refer to the next chapter and sections to understand the interpretation of your SHRP Score. You can then explore more effective ways to enhance it.

It is imperative to understand your SHRP SCORE. By discovering and implementing strategies to improve this score, individuals with chronic pain manage their wind-up effect and control of their bodies and minds, leading to a more fulfilling and satisfying life."

-Glenn Banks

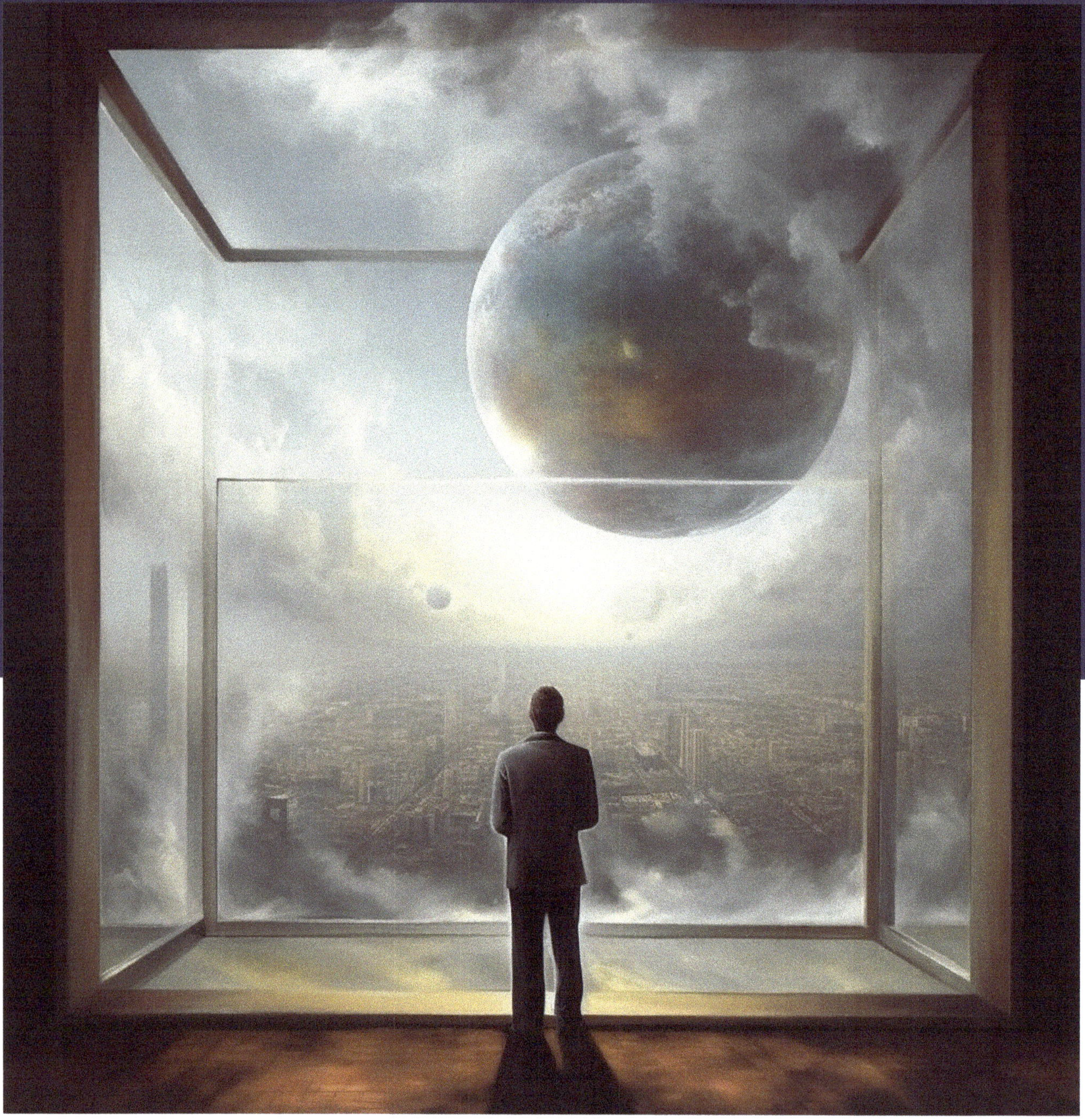

Chapter Fourteen

Exploring a Vision

To effectively manage chronic pain, focus on fulfilling your human needs in those five key areas. These include spirituality, belonging, variety, importance, and basic needs. Addressing these needs reduces the wind-up effect in your brain and improves your overall wellness.

In addition to medical, behavioral, and physical therapies outlined in the SHRP plan, addressing these fundamental human needs can provide a solid foundation for attaining wellness and managing chronic pain. Research has shown that addressing these needs can improve the quality of life and reduce the impact of chronic pain [83]

To monitor your progress and better understand your current chronic pain state, it's now essential to understand the Stages of Change model. Developed by psychologists James Prochaska and Carlo DiClemente, this model outlines the different stages individuals go through when undergoing behavioral change.[84]

Understanding these stages can help individuals and healthcare professionals identify where patients are in their ability to increase their SHRP Score, identify challenges they may be facing, and develop effective strategies to improve their overall wellness and manage chronic pain.

The Stages of Change Model is an essential tool for understanding complex and dynamic processes for behavioral change. This model outlines different stages individuals undergo when attempting to change their behavior [85]

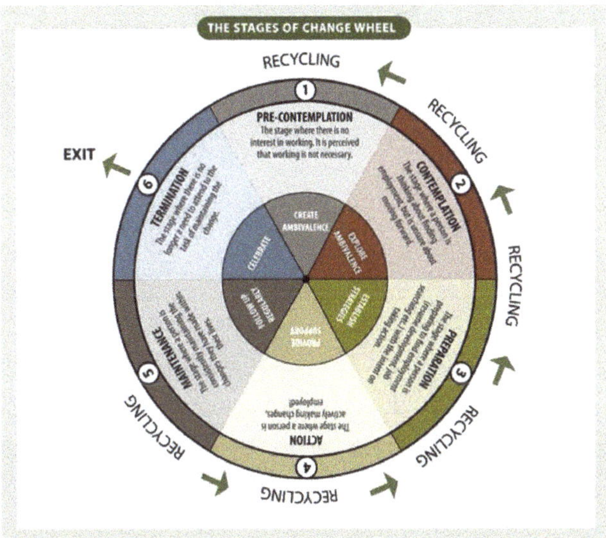

For instance, someone in the pre-contemplation stage may require education and information about the benefits of changing their behavior. Someone in the preparation stage may need assistance developing a concrete plan for change. The Stages of Change model recognizes that behavioral change involves various factors, such as motivation, social support, and self-efficacy.[86]

Individuals and professionals can benefit greatly by acquiring a comprehensive understanding of the complex nature of behavior change and the ability to recognize the different stages of change, especially when interacting with individuals with chronic pain.

This understanding enables them to approach a patient's change process with greater empathy, sensitivity, and efficacy. Moreover, it facilitates the identification of the patient's current stage of change, any barriers they may encounter, and the most suitable strategies to overcome them.

The Stages of Change Model consists of six stages, which are outlined as follows:

1. ***Pre-Contemplation:*** In this stage, individuals may or may not consider changing their behavior. They may be unaware of the need to change, or they may be resistant to the idea.

Some common statements made by Pre-Contemplative individuals may include:

- "I don't see any reason to change what I'm doing."
- "I don't think my behavior is a problem."
- "I don't have time to make any changes right now."
- "I'm too old/young to make changes."
- "I've tried before, and it didn't work."
- "I don't think I have the willpower to make any changes."
- "Other people have it worse than me."
- "I'm not interested in changing my behavior."
- "I'm too set in my ways to change."

2. ***Contemplation:*** In this stage, individuals consider changing their behavior but have not yet acted. They may be weighing the pros and cons of changing and determining if it is the right decision for them.

Some common statements made by Contemplative stage individuals may include:

- "I know I need to change, but I'm unsure how to do it."
- "I can see the benefits of changing, but it's hard to take the first step."
- "I'm worried about the challenges I'll face if I try to change."
- "I'm still weighing the pros and cons of changing."
- "I need more information before I can commit to making a change."
- "I'm thinking about making a change, but I'm not quite ready yet."
- "I'm not sure I have the confidence to make a change."

- "I'm considering making a change, but I'm worried about how it will affect others around me."

3. ***Preparation:*** In this stage, individuals have decided to change their behavior and plan to do so. They may be seeking support from others, gathering resources, and making concrete plans for change.

Some common statements made by preparation stage individuals may include:

- "I have a plan to make the necessary changes."
- "I'm ready to start taking action towards my goal."
- "I've set a start date to begin my new behavior."
- "I'm gathering the resources I need to make the change."
- "I'm excited about the possibilities of the change I'm about to make."
- "I'm committed to making a change, and I am willing to put in the effort to achieve it."
- "I'm confident that I can successfully make this change."
- "I'm seeking support from others to help me make this change."

4. ***Action:*** In this stage, individuals are actively engaged in changing their behavior. They may be using new strategies, seeking support from others, and facing challenges along the way.

Some common statements made by action-stage individuals may include:

- "I'm actively implementing the changes I've planned."
- "I'm making progress towards my goal every day."
- "I'm working hard to establish new habits."
- "I'm monitoring my progress and making adjustments as necessary."
- "I'm proud of the changes I've already made."
- "I'm finding new ways to stay motivated and committed to my goal."
- "I'm learning from my mistakes and using them as opportunities to improve."
- "I'm feeling more confident in my ability to sustain this change over time."

5. ***Maintenance:*** In this stage, individuals have successfully changed their behavior and are working to maintain their new habits. They may be seeking ongoing support and using strategies to prevent relapse.

Some common statements by maintenance stage individuals may include:

- "I've successfully integrated this new behavior into my life."
- "I'm continuing to practice the new behavior even though it's become routine."
- "I'm actively working to prevent relapse and stay on track."
- "I'm finding new ways to challenge myself and stay engaged with the behavior change."
- "I'm experiencing the benefits of the change, which motivates me to continue."
- "I'm sharing my success with others to inspire and encourage them to make changes too."
- "I'm celebrating my achievements and the progress I've made."
- "I'm still learning and growing as I maintain this change over time."

6. ***Termination:*** In this stage, individuals have successfully maintained their new behavior for an extended period, and it has become part of their normal routine. They may no longer need ongoing support or reminders to retain their new habits.

Some common statements by termination stage individuals may include:

- "I no longer engage in my old behavior."
- "I've completely replaced my old behavior with the new one."
- "The new behavior has become automatic, and I don't have to think about it anymore."
- "I'm confident I can maintain this behavior change for the rest of my life."
- "I don't feel like I'm missing out by not engaging in my old behavior."
- "I've developed new habits and routines that support the new behavior."
- "I'm no longer tempted to relapse into my old behavior."
- "I feel a sense of accomplishment and pride in myself for achieving this change."

It is important to acknowledge that the stages of change are not always experienced sequentially, and individuals may cycle through them sporadically. The key is to comprehend the underlying reasons for your current stage and how to facilitate progress towards the next stage.

"Change is a process, not an event. It takes time, energy, and commitment. Attempting to rush the process or skip stages can lead to frustration, setbacks, and ultimately, failure."

- Prochaska and DiClemente (1992)

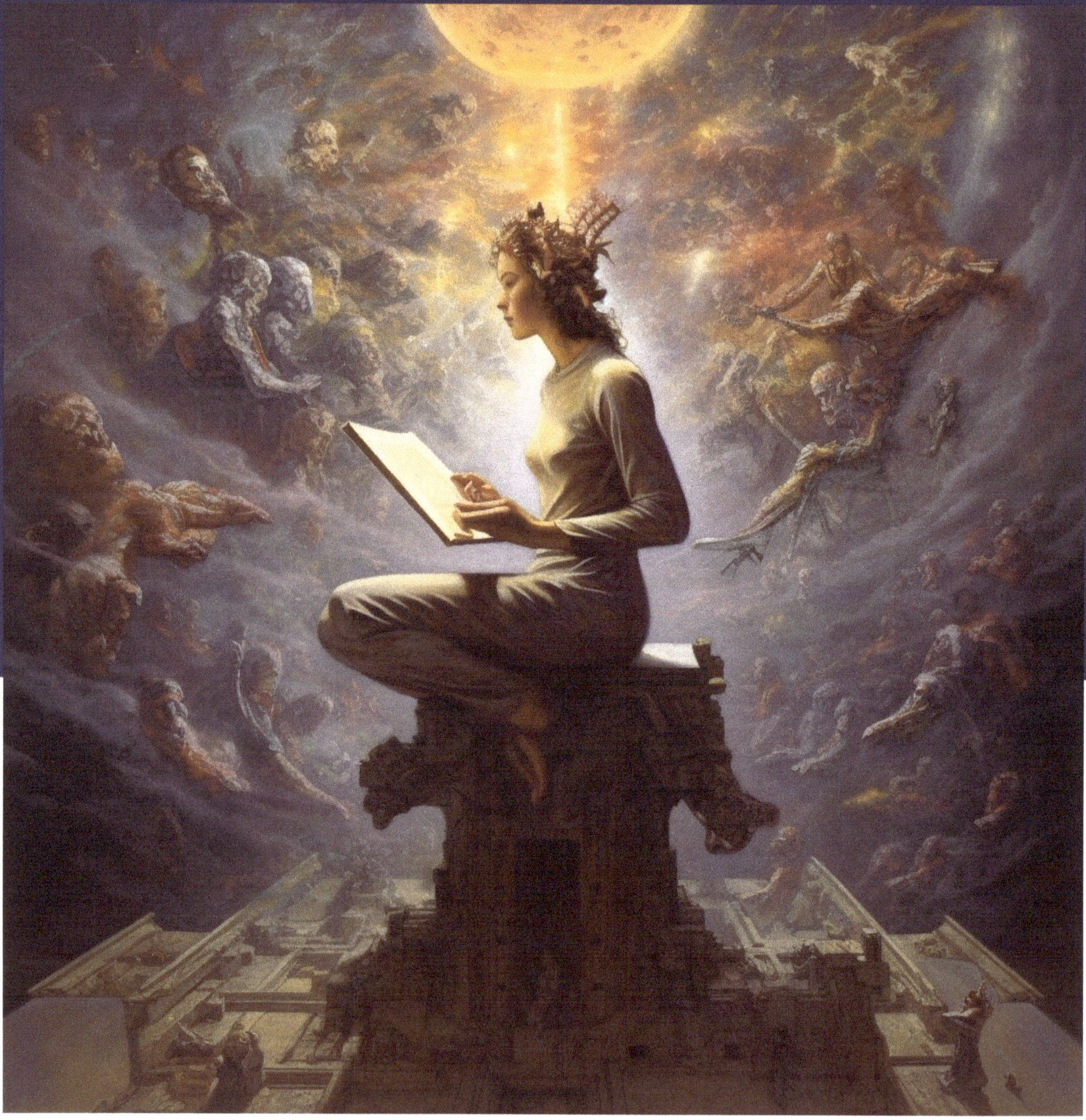

Chapter Fifteen

Determining Change

Individuals with chronic pain are encouraged to interpret and understand what stage of change they are in because it can help them identify where they are in the process of making behavioral changes related to their pain management.

By knowing which stage you are in, you can choose strategies that are more likely to be effective in helping you progress through the stages of change and ultimately achieve your goals.

As stated, if an individual is in the pre-contemplation stage, they may not yet see the need for change or be aware of the potential benefits of changing their pain management. In this case, interventions that increase awareness of the need for change, such as education about the risks of continued pain and the benefits of treatment, may be more effective than strategies that focus on developing action plans.

However, if a patient is in the action stage, they may benefit more from strategies that focus on maintaining motivation, managing setbacks, and developing coping skills.

By identifying their stage of change, patients can work with their family, friends, or healthcare providers to create a personalized plan of care tailored to their specific needs and goals. The following are the interpretations of your SHRP Score!

Record again your overall SHRP Score from Chapter 13 and compare it to the relevant stage listed below:

Your SHRP Score:

____

Termination Stage

If your score is between 45 and 50

As an individual with chronic pain, being in the termination stage of change would mean that you would have successfully integrated new behaviors and strategies into your daily life to manage chronic pain and have no desire to return to previous patterns of behavior. In other words, you have reached a point where the new behaviors have become habitual and are part of your everyday routine.[87]

Your wind-up effect is extremely low. It would mean your nervous system is less likely to become sensitized to pain. As a result, you may experience less pain intensity and duration than someone with a higher wind-up effect.

You may also have a higher pain threshold, meaning you can tolerate pain better. Additionally, you may not require as much pain medication or other pain management strategies as someone with a higher wind-up effect.

However, it's important to note that the wind-up effect is just one factor that contributes to chronic pain, and many other factors influence pain perception. Therefore, having a low wind-up effect does not guarantee that a person will be pain-free or won't require additional pain management strategies.

Here are some ways that a person in the termination stage of change could stay in that stage and maintain their progress:

- ***Celebrate success:*** Acknowledge and celebrate the progress made and the hard work put in to achieve the change. This can help build motivation to continue with the new behaviors and strategies.
- ***Reinforce new habits:*** Continue to reinforce the new habits and behaviors until they become fully automatic. This may involve setting up reminders, practicing positive self-talk, or enlisting social support.
- ***Develop a plan for relapse prevention:*** Identify potential triggers that could lead to a relapse and develop a plan to avoid or manage those triggers. This could involve seeking support from a therapist or support group, practicing stress-reduction techniques, or engaging in self-care activities.

- ***Continue to learn and grow:*** Seek out new information and resources to stay informed about the latest developments in chronic pain management and new coping strategies. This helps maintain motivation and prevent boredom or complacency.
- ***Be patient and persistent:*** Change is a process and setbacks may occur. Be patient and persistent in working towards long-term goals and maintaining progress.

Overall, being in the termination stage of change as a chronic pain patient is a significant accomplishment, and maintaining progress in this stage requires ongoing effort and commitment. By celebrating success, reinforcing new habits, developing a plan for relapse prevention, continuing to learn and grow, and being patient and persistent, individuals can stay in the termination stage and effectively manage chronic pain.

Maintenance Stage

If your score is between 40 and 44

As a chronic pain patient, being in the maintenance stage of change indicates that you have met many of your basic needs, but there is still room for improvement. This could mean that while you have access to basic physiological needs such as food, water, and shelter, you may still struggle with other needs like financial stability, social support, or access to healthcare.

According to the World Health Organization (WHO), basic human needs include physiological needs, safety and security, love and belongingness, esteem and self-worth, and self-actualization.[88]

Your score of 40 or more suggests that you have made progress toward meeting these needs. Areas of your life may need attention to manage your chronic pain effectively.

When an individual is in the stage of change characterized by a low, but not very low wind-up effect, it suggests that their nervous system is somewhat sensitive to pain, but less so than individuals with a higher wind-up effect. Although they may experience some pain intensity and duration, it may not be as severe as those with a higher wind-up effect.

Your pain threshold is moderate, meaning you tolerate some pain, but may require additional pain management strategies to manage it effectively. Although you may benefit from some pain medication or management techniques, you may not need as much as those with a higher wind-up effect.

It is important to remember that pain is a complex and subjective experience, and the wind-up effect is just one factor that can contribute to chronic pain. Other factors such as psychological and social factors influence pain perception and management.

Therefore, a person with a lower wind-up effect may still experience chronic pain and need additional pain management strategies.

If an individual in this stage has successfully changed their behavior, it is important to focus on sustaining their new habits over time. This can involve building a support system, utilizing positive reinforcement and support, and continuing to seek resources and tools to maintain their progress.

Action Stage

If your score is between 30 and 39

You are facing challenges in meeting some of your basic needs, which can have negative impacts on your physical and mental health. Depending on the specific needs that are not being met, you may be at risk of malnutrition, infectious diseases, mental health disorders, or other chronic health conditions.

Research has shown that individuals who experience poverty or socioeconomic disadvantage are more likely to have difficulty meeting their basic needs, which can further affect their health and ability to manage chronic pain.[89] Therefore, addressing social determinants of health such as poverty and inequality can be critical in improving overall health outcomes.

If an individual is in this middle stage of change, it suggests that their nervous system is moderately sensitive to pain. They may experience moderate pain intensity and duration. To manage their pain effectively, they may require a combination of medication, therapy, and other techniques.

Individuals with this level of wind-up effect may experience a range of emotions related to their pain, such as frustration, sadness, and anxiety. They may also have difficulty performing daily activities due to their pain.

Therefore, it's important for individuals with a wind-up effect in the middle to work with healthcare professionals to develop an individualized pain management plan that considers their specific needs and circumstances. This may involve a combination of medication, therapy, lifestyle changes, and other techniques to help manage their pain effectively and improve their quality of life.

If you are currently in this stage of change and working towards improving your situation, focus on utilizing new strategies and seeking support from others to overcome obstacles and maintain your motivation.

Preparation Stage

If your score is between 20 and 29

You face difficulty meeting your basic needs in different areas, such as food insecurity, lack of safe and stable housing, inadequate healthcare, or financial instability. You may also be experiencing mental health issues or social isolation, which adds to your stress and anxiety. Research has shown that unmet basic needs can increase perceived stress and risk of depression and anxiety disorders.[90]

For individuals who score low on the SHRP scale, meeting their basic needs and seeking resources and support to address their challenges is essential. This could mean accessing social services, seeking mental health support, or contacting community organizations.

If an individual is in the stage of change, their nervous system tends to be highly sensitive to pain, resulting in a more intense and enduring experience of pain compared to those with a lower wind-up effect. Furthermore, their pain threshold may be significantly lower, making it more challenging for them to withstand painful stimuli.

Due to their high wind-up effect, they may require increased pain management strategies to manage their pain effectively. These may include a combination of medication, physical therapy, and other techniques.

Individuals with a high wind-up effect may also experience emotional distress, such as depression, anxiety, and frustration, related to their chronic pain. They may struggle to engage in daily activities and may have difficulty sleeping due to their pain.

It's important to note that the wind-up effect is just one factor that contributes to chronic pain, and pain is a complex and subjective experience. Therefore, individuals with a high wind-up effect may benefit from working with healthcare professionals to create a personalized pain management plan that considers their needs and circumstances.

This may include a combination of treatments such as medication, cognitive-behavioral therapy, and other strategies to help manage their pain effectively and improve their quality of life.

You have decided to change your behavior and improve your score. Creating a specific change plan is essential. This involves setting achievable goals, identifying potential obstacles and solutions, and seeking resources and support to increase your SHRP Score.

Contemplative Stage

If your score is between 10 and 19

Your score on the SHRP Scale suggests a major deficiency in meeting your basic needs. This could be due to various factors such as poverty, homelessness, lack of access to healthcare or education, or other barriers preventing you from fulfilling your physiological and safety needs.

As a result, you may be experiencing significant levels of stress, anxiety, and physical discomfort, which can negatively impact your overall well-being and ability to manage your chronic pain.

Maslow's hierarchy of needs emphasizes that meeting physiological and safety needs is fundamental to achieving higher personal fulfillment and happiness.[91] Therefore, a low score on the SHRP scale could make it challenging to accomplish these higher-level needs.

If an individual is in this stage of change, their nervous system is sensitive to pain. As a result, they may experience severe and prolonged pain that can have a significant impact on their daily life. Their pain threshold may also be very low, making it difficult for them to tolerate even mild pain.

Due to their very high wind-up effect, they may require more aggressive pain management strategies to manage their pain effectively. These may include higher doses of medication, interventional pain procedures, physical therapy, and other techniques.

Individuals with a very high wind-up effect may also experience significant emotional distress, such as depression, anxiety, and frustration, related to their chronic pain. They may struggle to engage in daily activities and may have difficulty sleeping due to their pain.

It's important to note that the wind-up effect is just one factor that contributes to chronic pain, and pain is a complex and subjective experience. Therefore, individuals with a very high wind-up effect may benefit from working with healthcare professionals specializing in pain management to create a personalized plan that considers their needs and circumstances.

This may include a combination of treatments such as medication, cognitive-behavioral therapy, and other strategies to help manage their pain effectively and improve their quality of life.

If you are in this stage and considering changing your behavior, it helps to weigh the pros and cons of change and identify any barriers preventing you from acting. Seeking support from friends, family, or a professional can also aid in exploring your options and moving towards fulfilling your basic needs and better managing your chronic pain situation.

Pre-Contemplative Stage

If your score is between 0 and 9

It appears that you're currently facing multiple challenges in meeting any of your basic needs, which is leading to a range of physical, mental, and emotional difficulties. This situation is significantly impacting your ability to manage your chronic pain and wind-up effect.

You may be experiencing hunger, thirst, sleep deprivation, unsafe living conditions, or limited access to healthcare, which leaves you feeling overwhelmed, anxious, or stressed. It might be difficult to manage your day-to-day tasks and responsibilities.

Studies have shown that a lack of access to basic needs can have adverse effects on physical and mental health. For instance, insufficient sleep can impair cognitive function, and hunger can lead to malnutrition and various health issues. According to research published in the journal Social Science & Medicine, food and nutrition insecurity, a common experience among those who struggle to meet their basic needs, was linked to higher levels of stress and depression.[92]

When an individual's wind-up effect has reached the highest level, it indicates that their nervous system is extremely sensitive to pain signals. This can result in the experience of intense and prolonged pain, which may significantly impact their quality of life, even with minimal physical stimulation. Such individuals may also have a very low pain threshold, making it difficult for them to tolerate even mild pain.

Individuals with the highest possible wind-up effect require a multidisciplinary approach to pain management, which may include a combination of medication, physical therapy, psychological interventions, and lifestyle modifications. They may also benefit from alternative interventions such as acupuncture, massage, and relaxation techniques to help initially manage their chronic pain.

These individuals need to work closely with healthcare professionals to develop an extensive pain management plan and seek support from family and friends to help cope with the challenges of chronic pain. They may also benefit from connecting with support groups or seeking professional counseling to manage the emotional and psychological impact of living with chronic pain.

For individuals in the pre-contemplation stage, raising their awareness of the potential advantages of increasing their SHRP Score is important. This can involve providing information about the negative consequences of their current situation, such as experiencing stable or worsening pain, and exploring the positive outcomes of making a change, such as managing their chronic pain effectively.

After gaining a better understanding of their stage of change and the necessary techniques for self-motivation to facilitate behavioral changes for managing chronic pain, the individual can now shift their focus toward successfully implementing the SHRP approach.

> *"Believe in yourself and all that you are. Know that there is something inside you that is greater than any obstacle."*

-Christian Larson

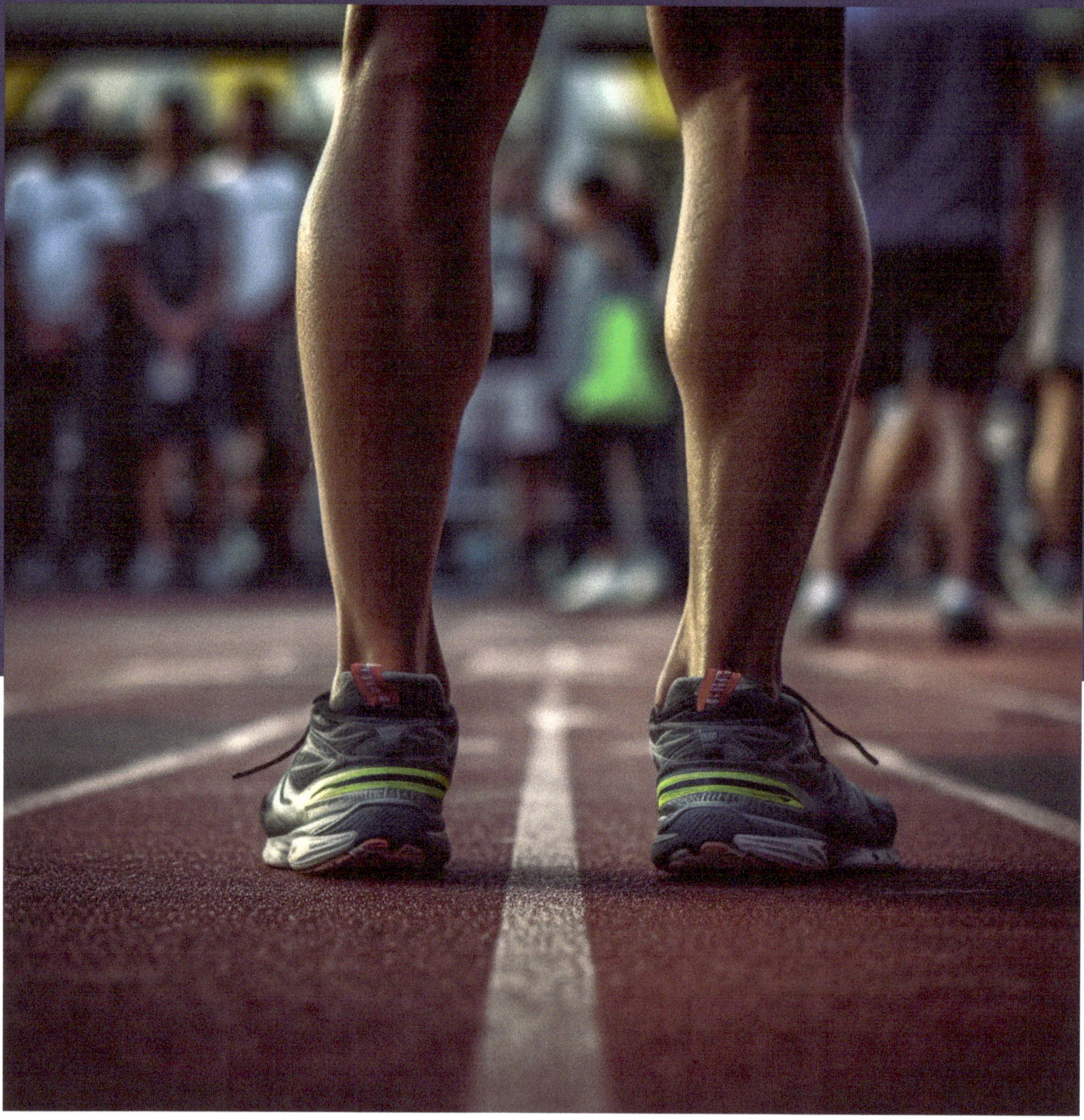

Chapter Sixteen

Desensitization Phases

The quote by Christian Larson highlights the human capacity to achieve great things, even in the face of adversity such as chronic pain, by believing in oneself and inner strength. By building self-confidence, individuals can overcome obstacles and achieve their goals.

The Strategic Harm Reduction Plan (SHRP) provides a structured approach to managing chronic pain and addressing key needs. It empowers individuals to take control of their situation and focus on critical areas to achieve a more fulfilling life. It may seem daunting initially, but even small steps significantly impact. Starting somewhere and moving forward is vital.

To determine which unmet needs require immediate attention, focus on the stage of change with the lowest score on the SHRP scale. By addressing these needs systematically, individuals can develop a sense of control and empowerment over their chronic pain situation, which can lead to quick and improved management of symptoms.

Research supports the use of the SHRP approach in managing chronic pain. A study published in the Journal of Pain Research found that addressing basic needs using a similar tool led to significant improvements in pain intensity, pain interference, depression, anxiety, and sleep disturbance in individuals with chronic pain.[93]

Another study published in the Journal of Pain found that addressing basic needs, such as sleep and social connection, in addition to medical treatment, led to improved pain management and decreased healthcare utilization.[94]

Following a complete understanding of their stage of change to manage chronic pain and mitigate the wind-up effect, the next step entails elevating the SHRP Score by successfully navigating the desensitization phases. This entails systematically addressing specific requisites, prioritizing them, and incorporating the desensitization techniques described below.

By doing so, individuals can exert greater control over their pain and promptly establish a sense of security, resulting in noteworthy enhancements in pain management as documented by empirical evidence.

The Desensitization Phases

Don't be discouraged by the idea of the desensitization process! This powerful process reduces the wind-up effect and manages chronic pain. It involves taking small, safe steps to gradually expose yourself to things that trigger your pain response.

You'll start with less intense stimuli and work your way up, allowing your brain to feel safe and build tolerance over time.

Remember, you don't need a pain management professional overseeing the process. While having a coach can be helpful, it's not necessary. Think of it like training for a physical goal - having a coach can make it easier, but ultimately, you have the power to achieve your goals on your own.

The desensitization process includes techniques like graded exposure therapy, cognitive-behavioral therapy, and mindfulness-based stress reduction.[95]

Start with the beginner phase and gradually work up to the expert and master phases outlined below. You can control and manage your pain and improve your quality of life.

Don't give up - you've got this!

Beginner Desensitization Phase

With the following proven techniques, you don't have to let chronic pain control your life any longer! Even if you're a novice, incorporating them can help you take back control of your chronic pain.

First, try incorporating breathing techniques like the Wim Hof method or "4444 method" into your daily routine. These methods help increase oxygen levels in your body, which can reduce pain and promote healing.

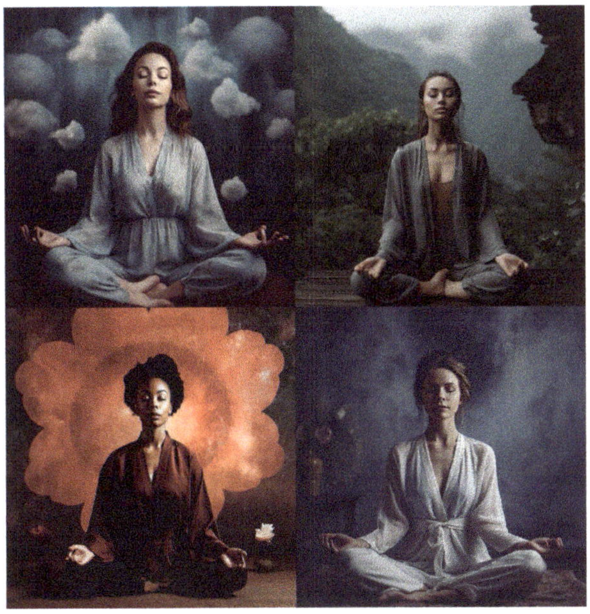

Next, practice mindfulness through meditation or using apps like Calm. These practices help calm the nervous system, reduce stress, and promote relaxation. Don't let chronic pain discourage you from exercising! Instead, try gentle exercise options like aqua therapy or "sit and be fit" programs. These exercises can improve your strength, flexibility, and overall well-being.

Gratitude is also a powerful tool for managing chronic pain. By acknowledging and expressing gratitude in your pain journal for the positive aspects of your life, you can release emotions and trigger protective brain chemicals that reduce pain.

Lastly, it's essential to understand the biology of chronic pain and how it affects your body. By gaining knowledge about the underlying mechanisms of chronic pain, you can better manage and control your pain.

Remember, you have the power to take control of your pain and "wind yourself down". Incorporate these techniques into your daily routine and see the positive changes for yourself. This is not a race; it is a lifestyle change.

Notes:

Expert Desensitization Phase

It's fascinating to note that managing chronic pain doesn't require moving to the wilderness and creating your sanctuary. You have successfully navigated the novice phase and achieved progress in managing your chronic pain, with noticeable improvements in your pain threshold. It's time to take your skills to the next level and become an expert in managing chronic pain.

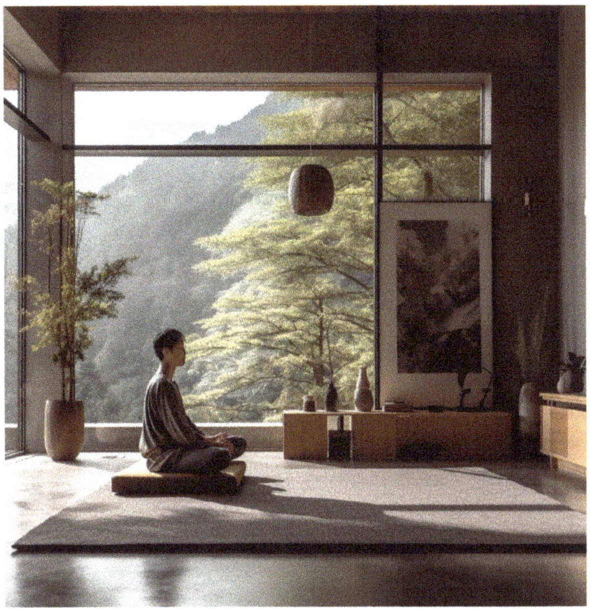

Incorporating the following practices into your daily routine takes your symptom management to the next level and dramatically reduces the wind-up effect.

It's important to distinguish between dependence on medication for pain management versus addiction. Understanding the difference can help you make informed decisions about your pain management plan and avoid potential addiction issues. With the right tools and approach, you can take control of your pain.

Next, address any depression or anxiety you may be experiencing by exploring the use of safety mechanisms to manage negative emotions and answer life questions. Don't be afraid to seek help from a mental health professional.

Simplify your life by decluttering your mind and focusing on your goals and direction. This can help you clarify what's important and reduce stress.

Finally, don't let social isolation and loneliness exacerbate your pain. Push back against these feelings by expanding your social boundaries, joining a support group, or reaching out to friends and family. Remember, you're not alone in your journey. A few simple changes control your pain.

Notes:

Master Desensitization Phase

You realize that managing chronic pain doesn't necessitate becoming a Zen Monk to experience the advantages. Your commendable progress in managing chronic pain has led to significant improvements. It's time to take your control to the next level and master your life's circumstances.

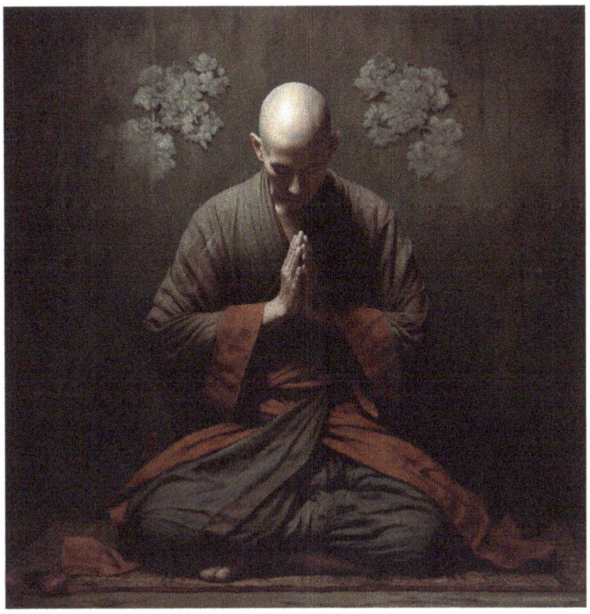

By incorporating some of the following techniques into your daily routine, you can continue to effectively manage your symptoms and enhance your quality of life meaningfully. Don't settle for just getting by when you can thrive with these proven practices.

Start by exploring how to use anger healthily to get your needs met without exacerbating your pain. Next, focus on building resilience to stress and managing adversity to reduce the impact of chronic pain on your mental and emotional health.

Begin by focusing on your nutrition and adding non-inflammatory supplements to your diet. This will support your overall health and reduce inflammation, which can exacerbate your pain.

Finally, identifying and addressing subconscious triggers related to past trauma is also crucial for managing chronic pain. Trauma can have a significant impact on the nervous system and can exacerbate pain symptoms. Addressing these triggers reduces their control of your daily life.

Notes:

"Take the first step in faith. You don't have to see the whole staircase, just take the first step."

-Martin Luther King Jr.

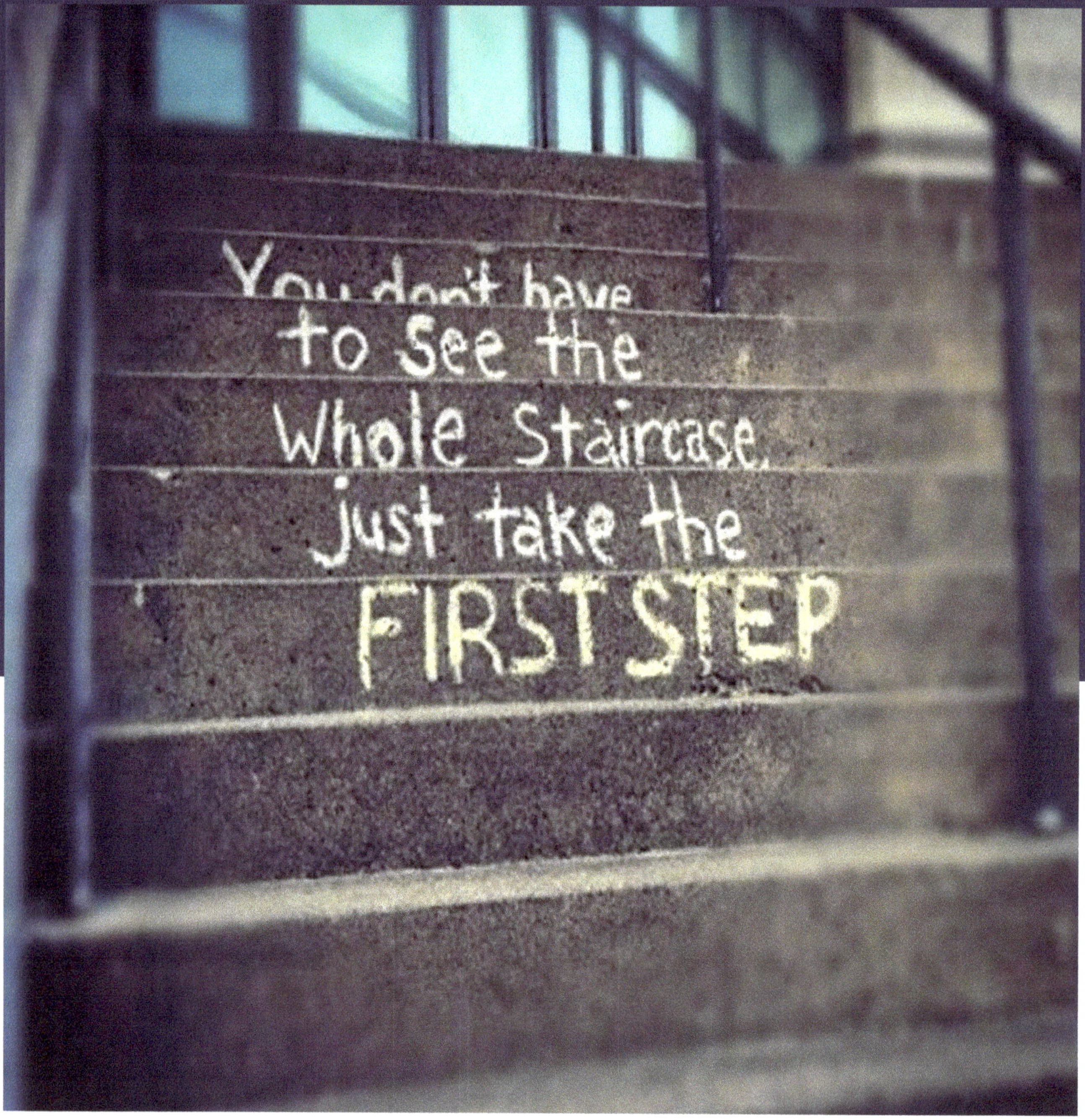

Chapter Seventeen

First Step

Here are the recommended steps to successfully implement the SHRP Approach:

- One helpful suggestion is to purchase a notebook and use it to keep track of your "creative tension," which includes your current reality, vision, and pain management goals. Consistently updating the notebook will allow you to monitor your progress and identify the slightest changes in meeting your human needs.
- Continue exploring your SHRP Score from Chapter Thirteen. Dedicate time for weekly introspection and gain a more profound understanding of how to enhance it.
- Research your current Stage of Change online and implement simple strategies to advance to the next stage.
- It is advisable to acquaint oneself with and progress through the Desensitization Phases, starting with the Beginner Phase and gradually advancing toward the Master Desensitization Phase. It is important to note that progress need not be rushed, as one can integrate one or two techniques at a time into a daily routine to ensure steady progress.

Incorporating desensitization techniques and following the SHRP Approach daily leads to incredible, evidence-based benefits that can significantly improve your quality of life.

This is possible because you are reaping the following benefits. You are rewiring your brain with trauma neural-plasticity remedies, regulating your CNS, reducing inflammation, and providing essential nutrients like magnesium, potassium, calcium, and oxygen.

But it doesn't stop there - these techniques also help combat boredom, loneliness, and isolation by encouraging social engagement and expanding your social networks.

You'll learn how to create a sense of safety in your brain, reducing anxiety, while also addressing negative thought patterns and behaviors that can interfere with pain management.

Ultimately, you'll take back control and function at the highest possible level, while meeting your basic needs, and finding a sense of belonging, variety, and importance along the way.

It's amazing what adding a few simple techniques can do for your overall well-being and management of chronic pain!

"Strength does not come from physical capacity. It comes from an indomitable will."

-Mahatma Gandhi

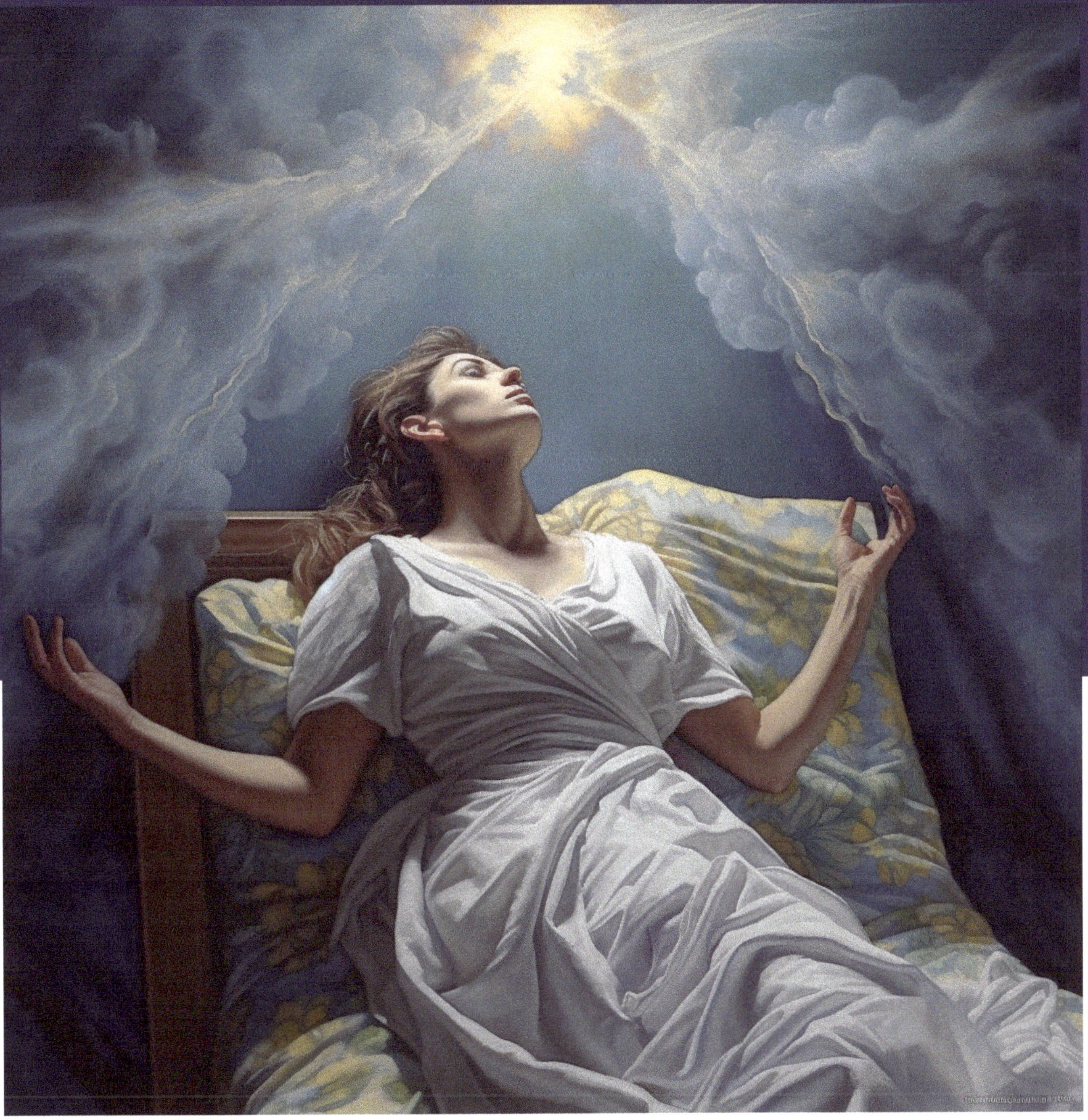

EPILOGUE

Hope & Encouragement

Living with chronic pain can be a challenging experience that affects millions of people around the world.[96] Chronic pain impacts physical and emotional well-being, social and occupational functioning, and overall quality of life.[97]

In this difficult journey, individuals with chronic pain require continuous encouragement and hope to manage their symptoms and improve their lives.[98]

Healthcare providers support chronic pain patients by continually providing messages of hope and motivation. Acknowledging the difficulties that chronic pain brings and encouraging patients to keep moving forward helps them maintain a positive outlook, focus on their goals, and stick to the plan.

Although chronic pain can be a challenging condition, it is manageable, and there is hope for a better quality of life.[99] Evidence-based interventions, including pharmacological, physical, cognitive-behavioral, and interventional therapies, effectively manage chronic pain and improve outcomes.[100]

Effective pain management makes a significant difference in improving the quality of life and reducing disability for those affected by chronic pain. Seeking support from loved ones or professional resources like therapists, social workers, or community organizations is invaluable in meeting these needs.

"It is essential to recognize that everyone has the fundamental right to meet their basic needs, and resources are available to help facilitate access to them."

-Glenn Banks

Remember that progress takes time and effort, but don't lose hope! With persistence, time, and support, you will improve your current situation and raise your SHRP Score. Healthcare providers are an important source of motivation and positivity, as patients who receive encouragement tend to be more committed to their treatment plans.

Take charge of your chronic pain by using the Strategic Harm Reduction Plan to continually identify your needs and develop a sense of current reality and vision.

It won't be easy, but the journey will be inspiring and empowering. By thinking creatively and overcoming obstacles, you will gradually reduce the impact of pain on your life and feel more in control.

So, keep believing in yourself and take that first step towards a brighter future. With determination and support, you overcome chronic pain and achieve your goals.

Resources

[1] Smith, S. M., Dart, R. C., & Katz, N. P. (2018). Challenges and opportunities in pain management in the context of the opioid epidemic. *Journal of addiction medicine, 12*(4), 255-262.

[2] McPherson, M. L., & Smith, M. B. (2019). Chronic pain management: navigating clinical, therapeutic, and systems challenges. *Journal of general internal medicine,* 34(12), 2674-2680.

[3] Institute of Medicine (US) Committee on Advancing Pain Research, Care, and Education. (2011). *Relieving pain in America: a blueprint for transforming prevention, care, education, and research.* National Academies Press (US).

[4] Merskey H, Bogduk N. *Classification of Chronic Pain: Descriptions of Chronic Pain Syndromes and Definitions of Pain Terms.* International Association for the Study of Pain. 1994.

[5] Woolf CJ. *Central sensitization: Implications for the diagnosis and treatment of pain.* Pain. 2011;152(3 Suppl): S2-S15. doi:10.1016/j.pain. 2010.09.030.

[6] Alshelh, Z., Di Pietro, F., Youssef, A. M., Reeves, J. M., Macey, P. M., Vickers, E. R., Peck, C. C., Murray, G. M., & Henderson, L. A. (2018). Chronic neuropathic pain: It's about the rhythm. *The Journal of Neuroscience,* 38(36), 7296-7304. doi: 10.1523/ JNEUROSCI.0300-18.201.

[7] Institute of Medicine. (2011). *Relieving pain in America: A blueprint for transforming prevention, care, education, and research.* The National Academies Press.

[8] Darnall BD, Stacey BR, Chou R. *Medical and psychological risks and consequences of long-term opioid therapy in women.* J Gen Intern Med. 2018 Dec;27(12):1673-81. doi: 10.1007/s11606-012-2185-1. Epub 2012 Jul 24. PMID: 22825826; PMCID: PMC3509336.

[9] Dowell D, Haegerich TM, Chou R. *CDC Guideline for Prescribing Opioids for Chronic Pain - United States,* 2016. MMWR Recomm Rep. 2016 Mar 18;65(1):1-49. doi: 10.15585/mmwr.rr6501e1. PMID: 26987082.

[10] Louw A, Diener I, Landers M, et al. *Barriers and facilitators to the implementation of evidence-based chronic pain management in primary care: a qualitative study of patients and providers. Pain Pract.* 2017;17(6):782-791. doi:10.1111/papr.1254.

[11} Darnall BD, Mackey SC, Lorig K, et al. *Comparative effectiveness of cognitive behavioral therapy for chronic pain and chronic pain self-management within the context of voluntary patient-centered prescription opioid tapering: The EMPOWER study protocol.* Pain Med. 2019;20(10):1919-1929. doi:10.1093/pm/pnz144.

[12] St. Marie BJ, Williams LS. *Management of chronic pain in primary care.* In: Benzon HT, Raja SN, Liu SS, Fishman SM, Cohen SP (eds). Essentials of Pain Medicine (Fourth Edition). Elsevier. 2018:389-397.

[13] Upshur CC, Luckmann RS, Savageau JA. *Primary care provider concerns about management of chronic pain in community clinic populations.* J Gen Intern Med. 2006;21(6):652-655. doi:10.1111/j.1525-1497.2006.00468.

[14]] Centers for Disease Control and Prevention (CDC). (2019). *The prescription opioid overdose epidemic: an overview.* https://www.cdc.gov/drugoverdose/epidemic/index.html.

[15] Centers for Disease Control and Prevention. (2019). *Online Training Series. Retrieved* from https://www.cdc.gov/drugoverdose/training/nonopioid/index.html.

[16] Association of American Medical Colleges. (2021). *Pain Management Education.* Retrieved from https://www.aamc.org/what-we-do/mission-areas/medical-education/medical-education-issues/pain-management-education.

[17] Veterans Health Administration. (2021). *National Pain Management Strategy.* Retrieved from https://www.va.gov/PAINMANAGEMENT/nationalpainmanagementstrategy.asp.

[18] American Physical Therapy Association. (2021). *Pain Management.* Retrieved from https://www.apta.org/patient-care/pain-management.

[19] Centers for Disease Control and Prevention. (2018). *The CDC Guideline for Prescribing Opioids for Chronic Pain.* Retrieved from https://www.cdc.gov/drugoverdose/prescribing/guideline.html.

[20] Centers for Disease Control and Prevention. (2018). *Prescription Drug Overdose: Prevention for States.* Retrieved from https://www.cdc.gov/drugoverdose/states/state_prevention.html.

[21] Centers for Disease Control and Prevention. (2019). *Online Training Series.* Retrieved from https://www.cdc.gov/drugoverdose/training/nonopioid/index.html.

[22] Association of American Medical Colleges. (2021). *Pain Management Education.* Retrieved from https://www.aamc.org/what-we-do/mission-areas/medical-education/medical-education-issues/pain-management-education.

[23] American Physical Therapy Association. (2021). *Pain Management.* Retrieved from https://www.apta.org/patient-care/pain-management.

[24] National Institutes of Health. (2021). *Pain Management.* Retrieved from https://nccih.nih.gov/health/pain.

[25] Kimbrell, T., Edwards, C. L., Mardekian, J., Staud, R., Kairys, A., & Sikes, K. A. (2019). *Association of a single-session educational intervention with compliance and outcomes in individuals with chronic pain.* Journal of Pain Research, 12, 153-161. doi: 10.2147/JPR.S179814.

[26] Watt-Watson, J., McGillion, M., Hunter, J., Choiniere, M., Clark, A. J., Dewar, A., . . . Webber, K. (2016). *A survey of prelicensure pain curricula in health science faculties in Canadian universities. Pain Research & Management,* 2016, 1-9. doi:10.1155/2016/6958932.

[27] Kerns, R. D., Burns, J. W., Shulman, M., Jensen, M. P., Nielson, W. R., Czlapinski, R., . . . Dallas, M. I. (2019). *Can we improve cognitive–behavioral therapy for chronic back pain treatment engagement and adherence? Results from a randomized controlled trial. Pain,* 160(11), 2569-2577. doi:10.1097/j.pain.0000000000001639.

[28] Keefe, F. J., Abernethy, A. P., C Campbell, L., & Main, C. J. (2019). *Psychological approaches to understanding and treating pain. Annual Review of Psychology,* 70, 201-225. doi:10.1146/annurev-psych-010418-102901Note: Here are the primary sources related to the major benefits of neuropsychological education in chronic pain management and combating stigma.

[29] Singh, J., & Sloan, M. (2022). *The biopsychosocial model of chronic pain: A review of its application in the management of chronic spinal pain.* Current Reviews in Musculoskeletal Medicine, 15(3), 331-341. doi: 10.1007/s12178-022-09660-w.

[30] Gatchel, R.J., & Mayer, T.G. (2019). *Evidence-informed management of chronic low back pain with the biopsychosocial* (BPS) model. Neuropsychology Review, 29(1), 49-60. doi: 10.1007/s11065-018-9385-x.

[31] Dowell, D., Haegerich, T.M., & Chou, R. (2016). *CDC guideline for prescribing opioids for chronic pain — United States,* 2016. JAMA, 315(15), 1624-1645. doi: 10.1001/jama.2016.1464.

[32] Asmundson, G. J. G., Coons, M. J., Taylor, S., & Katz, J. (2004). PTSD and the experience of pain: research and clinical implications of shared vulnerability and mutual maintenance models. **Journal of traumatic stress**, 17(4), 299-309.(2) Heinberg, L. J.,

[33] Kudel, I., White, M. A., & de Zwaan, M. (2006). *Assessment of body image concerns in obese patients with binge eating disorder. Obesity surgery*, 16(9), 1199-1204.

[34] Tietjen, G. E., Brandes, J. L., Peterlin, B. L., Eloff, A., Dafer, R. M., & Stein, M. R. (2015). Childhood maltreatment and migraine (part I). Prevalence and adult revictimization: a multicenter headache clinic survey. Headache: *The Journal of Head and Face Pain*, 55(5), 819-832.

[35] Guille, C., Nentwich, L., Heilbron, N., & McLaughlin, J. (2018). *Trauma-informed care in medical education: current knowledge and future directions.* Academic Psychiatry, 42(1), 82-85.

[36] 1 Woolf, C. J. (2011). *Central sensitization: implications for the diagnosis and treatment of pain.* Pain, 152(3 Suppl), S2-S15. doi: 10.1016/j.pain.2010.09.030.

[37] Baliki, M. N., Geha, P. Y., Apkarian, A. V., & Chialvo, D. R. (2008). Beyond feeling chronic pain hurts the brain, disrupting the default-mode network dynamics. *Journal of Neuroscience*, 28(6), 1398-1403.

[38] Davis, K. D., Moayedi, M., & Taylor, K. S. (2017). *Brain imaging in chronic pain: the state of the art.* Nature Reviews Neurology, 13(11), 627-638.

[39] Woolf, C. J. (2011). *Central sensitization: implications for the diagnosis and treatment of pain.* Pain, 152(3), S2-S15.

[40] Lenz, F. A., Rios, M., Chau, D., & Krauss, G. (1993). Persistent pain after spinal cord injury is maintained by primary afferent input. *Journal of Neuroscience*, 13(2), 799-812.

[41] Woolf, C. J., & Salter, M. W. (2000). *Neuronal plasticity: increasing the gain in pain.* Science, 288(5472), 1765-1769.

[42] Dowell, D., Haegerich, T. M., & Chou, R. (2016). CDC guideline for prescribing opioids for chronic pain—United States, 2016. JAMA, 315(15), 1624-1645.

[43a] Vachon-Presseau, E., Tétreault, P., Petre, B., Huang, L., Berger, S. E., Torbey, S., ... & Jackson, P. L. (2016). *Corticolimbic anatomical characteristics predetermine risk for chronic pain.* Brain, 139(7), 1958-1970. doi: 10.1093/brain/aww10.

[43b] Baliki, M. N., Schnitzer, T. J., Bauer, W. R., & Apkarian, A. V. (2011). *Brain morphological signatures for chronic pain.* PLoS ONE, 6(10), e26010. doi: 10.1371/journal.pone.0026010.

[43c] Tracey, I., & Bushnell, M. C. (2009). How neuroimaging studies have challenged us to rethink: Is chronic pain a disease? *The Journal of Pain*, 10(11), 1113-1120. doi: 10.1016/j.jpain.2009.06.012.

[43d] Pinto, P. R., McIntyre, T., Ferrero, R., Almeida, A., Araújo-Soares, V., & Jensen, M. P. (2019). *Predicting chronic pain outcomes using pain intensity as a predictor.* Pain, 160(3), 662-669. doi: 10.1097/j.pain.0000000000001441.

[44] Flor, H. (2008). *Maladaptive plasticity, memory for pain and phantom limb pain: review and suggestions for new therapies.* Expert review of neurotherapeutics, 8(5), 809-818.

[45] Apkarian, A. V., Baliki, M. N., & Farmer, M. A. (2013). *Predicting transition to chronic pain.* Current opinion in neurology, 26(4), 360-367.

[46] Ezzatian-Ahar, J., Babaei-Ghazani, A., Ghorbani, Z., Rezaei, M., & Nejati, V. (2021). *The effect of high-definition transcranial direct current stimulation on pain and function in patients with chronic knee osteoarthritis: a randomized double-blind sham-controlled trial. Pain*, 162(2), 512-519.

[47] Zeidan, F., Emerson, N. M., Farris, S. R., Ray, J. N., Jung, Y., McHaffie, J. G., & Coghill, R. C. (2020). Mindfulness meditation-based pain relief employs different neural mechanisms than placebo and sham mindfulness meditation-induced analgesia. *Journal of Neuroscience*, 40(5), 1145-1157.

[48] Brungs, S., & Kelly, P. (2008). *Creating a safe and healthy healthcare environment.* HealthcarePapers, 8(SP), 68-72.

[49] Centers for Disease Control and Prevention. (n.d.). *Infection prevention in healthcare settings*. Retrieved from: https://www.cdc.gov/infectioncontrol/index.html.

[50] Joint Commission International. (n.d.). *International patient safety goals*. Retrieved from: https://www.jointcommissioninternational.org/standards/international-patient-safety-goals/.

[51] World Health Organization. (n.d.). *Patient safety curriculum guide: multi-professional edition*. Retrieved from https://www.who.int/patientsafety/education/mp_curriculum_guide/en/.

[52] Lerner JS, Gonzalez RM, Small DA, Fischhoff B. *Effects of fear and anger on perceived risks of terrorism: A national field experiment*. Psychological Science. 2003 Sep;14(5):144-50.

[53] Marazziti D, Palego L, Giannaccini G, Mungai F, Cassano GB. *Neurobiology of emotions*. Rivista di psichiatria. 2011 Sep;46(5):290-9.

[54] Northoff G, Boeker H, Richter A, Grimm S, Weniger G, Gass P, et al. Reduced activation and altered laterality in two neurocognitive systems during simple surgical pain in major depression. *Journal of psychiatric research*. 2005 May 1;39(3):245-57.

[55] Seasholtz AF, Valenzuela CF. Modulation of GABA-A *receptor function during development and following injury*. In International Review of Neurobiology 2001 Jan 1 (Vol. 46, pp. 263-283). Academic Press.

[56] *"Opioids are not the best medicine for chronic pain."* NBC News, 5 April 2023, https://www.nbcnews.com/health/health-news/opioids-are-not-best-medicine-chronic-pain-rcna20744. Accessed 20 April 2023.

[57] *"Why opioids are not the best medicine for chronic pain."* Harvard Health Blog, 22 March 2023, https://www.health.harvard.edu/blog/why-opioids-are-not-the-best-medicine-for-chronic-pain-2023032220459. Accessed 20 April 2023.

[58] *"Opioids not effective for chronic pain, new study confirms."* Medical News Today, 27 February 2023, https://www.medicalnewstoday.com/articles/opioids-not-effective-for-chronic-pain-new-study-confirms. Accessed 20 April 2023.

[59] Tolerance: "Opioid Tolerance and Dependence: A Clinical Perspective" - *Journal of Pain and Palliative Care Pharmacotherapy*, 2019.

[60] Dependence and addiction: "Opioid Addiction 2016 Facts and Figures" - American Society of Addiction Medicine, 2016; and *"Managing Chronic Pain with Opioids: A Call for Change"* - New England Journal of Medicine, 2019.

[61] Side effects: *"Opioids and the Management of Chronic Pain: Controversies, Current Status, and Future Directions"* - Expert Review of Clinical Pharmacology, 2019; and "Opioids for Chronic Pain: A Review of Guidelines and Recommendations" - Pain Research and Management, 2020.

[62] Overdose: *"Opioid Overdose Crisis"* - National Institute on Drug Abuse, 2021; and "Opioid Overdose Deaths by Type of Opioid" - Centers for Disease Control and Prevention, 2021.

[63] Alternative treatments: *"Non-opioid Pharmacologic Treatments for Chronic Pain"* - American Family Physician, 2018; and *"Physical Therapy Interventions for Chronic Pain"* - Physical Therapy, 2019.

[64] Koob, G. F., & Volkow, N. D. (2010). *Neurocircuitry of addiction. Neuro psycho pharmacology,* 35(1), 217-238.

[65] Nestler, E. J. (2013). Cellular basis of memory for addiction. *Dialogues in clinical neuroscience,* 15(4), 431-443.

[66] Koob, G. F., & Le Moal, M. (2001). *Drug addiction, dysregulation of reward, and allostasis.* Neuropsychopharmacology, 24(2), 97-129.

[67] American Psychiatric Association. (2013). *Diagnostic and statistical manual of mental disorders* (5th ed.). https://doi.org/10.1176/appi.books.9780890425596.

[68] World Health Organization. (2018). *International classification of diseases for mortality and morbidity statistics* (11th Revision). https://icd.who.int/browse11/l-m/en.

[69] National Institute on Drug Abuse. (2018). *Understanding drug use and addiction.* https://www.drugabuse.gov/publications/drugfacts/understanding-drug-use-addiction.

[70] Center for Substance Abuse Treatment. (2004). Chapter 2: *Definitions of Dependence and Addiction. Substance Abuse Treatment: Addressing the Specific Needs of Women.* US Department of Health and Human Services.

[71] National Institute on Drug Abuse. (2020). *Principles of Drug Addiction Treatment: A Research-Based Guide* (Third Edition). Drug Addiction Treatment in the United States.

[72] Volkow, N. D., & McLellan, A. T. (2016). Opioid abuse in chronic pain—misconceptions and mitigation strategies. *New England Journal of Medicine*, 374(13), 1253-1263.

[73] [1] Turk, D. C., & Okifuji, A. (2002). Psychological factors in chronic pain: evolution and revolution. *Journal of consulting and clinical psychology*, 70(3), 678.

[74] McCracken, L. M., & Iverson, G. L. (2001). Disrupted sleep patterns and daily functioning in patients with chronic pain. *Pain Research & Management*, 6(3), 137-142.

[75] Vlaeyen, J. W., & Linton, S. J. (2012). *Fear-avoidance and its consequences in chronic musculoskeletal pain: a state of the art. Pain*, 157(8), 1587-1590.

[76] Fritz, R. (1989). *The path of least resistance: Learning to become the creative force in your own life*. Ballantine Books.

[77] Gundersen, C., Hake, M., Dewey, A., Engelhard, E., & Crumbaugh, A. (2018). Food insecurity and anxiety in the United States: An analysis of the 2016 National Survey of Children's Health. *Journal of Social and Clinical Psychology*, 37(9), 666-687.

[78] National Law Center on Homelessness and Poverty. (2009). Homes not handcuffs: The criminalization of homelessness in U.S. cities. Retrieved from: https://nlchp.org/wp-content/uploads/2018/10/Homes-Not-Handcuffs-FINAL.pdf.

[79] Van der Kolk, B. (2014). *The body keeps the score: Brain, mind, and body in the healing of trauma*. Penguin Books.

[80] Graven-Nielsen, T., et al. (2002). Immobilization induces muscle hyperalgesia in healthy individuals. *The Journal of Pain*, 3(1), 28-37.

[81] Lu, Y., et al. (2012). *Immobilization induces changes in presynaptic control of group afferents in healthy humans.* Neuroscience Letters, 509(1), 36-40.

[82] Moseley, G. L. (2002). *Graded motor imagery is effective for long-standing complex regional pain syndrome: a randomized controlled trial*. Pain, 108(1-2), 192-198.

[83] Grönlund, A. S., Öhlén, J., & Ziegert, K. (2016). The impact of fulfilling the five basic needs on quality of life and subjective well-being. *Journal of Happiness Studies*, 17(6), 2455-2469. doi: 10.1007/s10902-015-9712-1.

[84] Prochaska, J. O., & DiClemente, C. C. (1982). *Transtheoretical therapy: Toward a more integrative model of change.* Psychotherapy: Theory, Research & Practice, 19(3), 276-288. doi: 10.1037/h0088437.

[85] Miller, W. R., & Rollnick, S. (2012). *Motivational interviewing: Helping people change* (3rd ed.). New York: Guilford Press.

[86] Velicer, W. F., Prochaska, J. O., Fava, J. L., Norman, G. J., & Redding, C. A. (1998). *Smoking cessation and stress management: Applications of the transtheoretical model of behavior change.* Homeostasis in Health and Disease, 38(5-6), 216-233.

[87] Prochaska, J. O., & DiClemente, C. C. (1984). *The transtheoretical approach: Crossing traditional boundaries of therapy.* Homewood, IL: Dow Jones/Irwin.

[88] World Health Organization. (2013). *Mental Health Action Plan* 2013-2020. Geneva, Switzerland: World Health Organization.

[89] Adler, N. E., & Stewart, J. (2010). *Health disparities across the lifespan: meaning, methods, and mechanisms.* Annals of the New York Academy of Sciences, 1186(1), 5-23.

[90] Zhang, W., Xu, J., Zhao, J., & Ye, M. (2017). Unmet basic needs as a chronic stressor underlying health disparities: *A systematic review and meta-review. Journal of Psychosomatic Research*, 103, 1-9. doi: 10.1016/j.jpsychores. 2017.09.008.

[91] 1 Maslow, A. H. (1943). *A theory of human motivation.* Psychological Review, 50(4), 370-396.

[92] Lee, H., Harris, K. M., & Lee, J. (2018). *Multiple dimensions of food insecurity and depressive symptoms among college students.* Social Science & Medicine, 214, 36-45. doi: 10.1016 j.socscimed.2018.08.033.

[93] Feliu-Soler, A., Montesinos, F., Gutiérrez-Martínez, O., Scott, W., McCracken, L. M., Luciano, J. V., & Peñarrubia-María, M. T. (2018). Current status of acceptance and commitment therapy for chronic pain: a narrative review. *Journal of pain research*, 11, 2145–2159. https://doi.org/10.2147/JPR.S154655..

[94] Gaskell, H., Derry, S., Stannard, C., & Moore, R. A. (2014). *Pain relief and side effects of painkillers: a longitudinal community study.* BMC Public Health, 14, 1–9. https://doi.org/10.1186/1471-2458-14-964.

[95] Scheman J. (2016). Desensitization for Chronic Pain. In Pain Management Secrets (4th ed., pp. 365-369). Elsevier. https://doi.org/10.1016/B978-0-323-34167-8.00042-1.

[96] American Academy of Pain Medicine. (2016). Facts and Figures on Pain. Retrieved from https://www.painmed.org/patient-center/facts-on-pain/.

[97] Institute of Medicine (US) Committee on Advancing Pain Research, Care, and Education. (2011). Relieving Pain in America: A Blueprint for Transforming Prevention, Care, Education, and Research. National Academies Press (US). https://www.ncbi.nlm.nih.gov/books/NBK92516/.

[98] Turk, D. C., Wilson, H. D., & Cahana, A. (2011). Treatment of chronic pain: Progress and future directions. Journal of pain, 12(7), 1-8. https://doi.org/10.1016/j.jpain.2011.02.002.

[99] Breivik, H., Collett, B., Ventafridda, V., Cohen, R., & Gallacher, D. (2006). Survey of chronic pain in Europe: prevalence, impact on daily life, and treatment. European journal of pain, 10(4), 287-333. https://doi.org/10.1016/j.ejpain.2005.06.009.

[100] Williams, A. C., Eccleston, C., & Morley, S. (2012). Psychological therapies for the management of chronic pain (excluding headache) in adults. Cochrane Database of Systematic Reviews, 11. https://doi.org/10.1002/14651858.CD007407.pub3.

www.ingramcontent.com/pod-product-compliance
Lightning Source LLC
LaVergne TN
LVHW071201210926
848482LV00014B/703